To June Baca,
Thank you for your
contribution to this
book, Marge Rieder

MILLBORO
AND MORE

Introducing Hypnotherapy for
Stroke Paralysis

MARGE RIEDER, Ph.D.

Blue Dolphin Publishing

Published by Blue Dolphin Publishing, Inc.
P.O. Box 8, Nevada City, CA 95959
Orders: 1-800-643-0765
Web: www.bluedolphinpublishing.com

ISBN: 1-57733-129-X

Library of Congress Cataloging-in-Publication Data

Rieder, Marge.
   Millboro, and more : introducing hypnotherapy for stroke paralysis /
Marge Rieder.
      p. cm.
Includes bibliographical references.
   ISBN 1-57733-129-X (pbk. : alk. paper)
   1. Rieder, Marge. 2. Reincarnation therapy—Popular works.
3. Cerebrovascular disease—Popular works. I. Title.

RC489.R43R53 2003
133.9'01'35—dc22

                                                     2003021798

Printed in the United States of America

10   9   8   7   6   5   4   3   2   1

This book is dedicated
to my daughter Evie
who has donated more time and input
to the Millboro story than any other one person.
It was Evie's character, "Running Springs,"
who stated that the Indians had built the kivas under Millboro.
Also she explained the interaction between the early settlers
in the Millboro area and the Indians that eventually
laid the background for the entire story.
M.R.

It is easier to ignore the obvious than to defy tradition.
Unknown

*There are more things in heaven and earth
than are dreamed of in your philosophy....*
Shakespeare

CONTENTS

1. Robin's Nest   1
   Warm Springs Inn   10
   Supplies for Gettysburg?   13

2. The Confederate White House   16

3. Millboro   23

4. The Big White Rock   32

5. Hypnosis   47

6. Controlling the Emotions with Hypnosis   56

7. Confidence   65

8. A Close Look at Homosexuality   77

9. Life in the Womb   87

10. Twin Study   102

11. Phantom Limb Pain   115

12. Spirit Releasment   121

13. Utilizing the Power of the Unconscious Mind   129

14. A Baby for Queen Christina   143

15. Stroke Strategy   **155**
    The Nervous System   159
    Ernie Adams   160
    Bob Jenkins   164
    Walter Hopp   166
    June Baca   166
    Ray Conniff   167
    Diane Bingham   169
    Madelina de Paz   171
    Secondary Gain   175
    Suggestions for Stroke Subjects   176

Afterword   178

Bibliography   182

You do something to me,
something that simply mystifies me.
Tell me, why should it be
You have the power to hypnotize me?

"You Do Something to Me" from the musical,
Fifty Million Frenchmen, 1929

CHAPTER ONE

ROBIN'S NEST

HIGH ON THE CREST OF THE MOUNTAIN above Millboro, Virginia, is the area that once was the Indian village of Robin's Nest. Following the only main road that leads out of Millboro, in the opposite direction from the county road, up over the mountain, one comes to the Indian village area. Continuing on the county road, over the crest and down the other side, the road terminates in an area of several homes called, strangely enough, Little California.

The site of Robin's Nest is at the very top of this mountain and is divided between two counties. One part is in Bath County and the other half is in Rockbridge. A large sign on the road, right at the entrance of Robin's Nest, denotes the county dividing line.

Three trails lead off to the right, as one comes up from Millboro, into the main area of the former village. The center trail goes directly to the living area—three very large meadows, each surrounded on three sides by tall privet hedges. The trail off to the right runs directly along the back of the compound and terminates suddenly.

Branching off to the left (from the county highway entrance) a third trail takes one back, away from the heart of the camp to a large circular cleared area. This we have dubbed the "pow-wow" area, as one can almost see the huge bonfire in the center as the tribal braves conduct a ritual ceremonial dance.

Heading in the opposite direction from the main highway, to the left, a large trail leads back into the woods. On my first visit to the area I walked a mile or so along this path. Coming on a rather flat area, I was surprised to find several rows of some type of grain growing.

Obviously at one time it had been a carefully tended crop area, reseeding itself yearly since the Indians had left there. Down the mountain about a hundred feet or so, I discovered a small, tranquil spring-fed pool of water, which undoubtedly was used to irrigate the crops above.

How nice it would be if some philanthropic organization would lease the Robin's Nest area and restore it, as the Rockefeller Foundation did at Williamsburg. It would not be difficult or expensive, as the grounds are intact and all that would be needed, primarily, would be teepees and wickiups. It would be interesting to children today who depend so on our electronically oriented society.

The fact of the still-growing crops was noted in my first book, *Mission to Millboro*. A year or so after release of the book, I went back to the crop area hoping to get pictures. I was shocked to see the whole growing area had been plowed under—there was no trace of the growing crops.

The people of Millboro were interested, to varying degrees, in the development of this story as it progressed. That is, until Fox Television released the *Sightings* show featuring the Millboro story. The show explained how one of the people in the story had told of a hidden room under "Grandma's" house that was used to hide escaping slaves. She had marked an "X" on Grandma's house in a photo of the old town taken shortly after the Civil War. While the *Sightings* group was in Millboro, we met up with the owner of the property who had dug a ditch next to the room and made a hole in the wall so we could see in. A spotlight, when shown into the room, revealed a large room exactly as it had been described to me.

It is my opinion that until that time most of the townspeople had not taken this work very seriously. Immediately after the *Sightings* segment aired, everyone's attitude changed abruptly. I have been

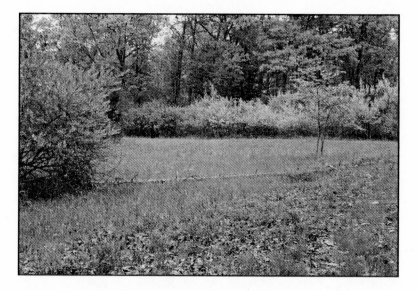

Living area of Robin's Nest

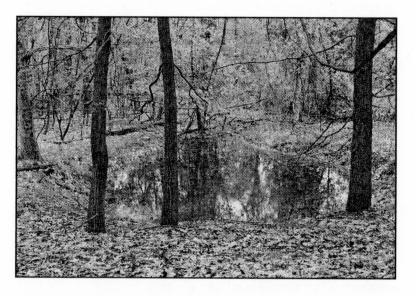

Small mountain pool used to water crops near Robin's Nest

told that the townspeople desperately do not wish to be overrun by curiosity-seekers. One woman said to me, "We don't want a bunch of archaeologists coming into town, tearing the place up." Others said that racism was a large factor. "We don't want a bunch of niggers coming into town, wanting to see where Grandma and Grandpa hid while they were escaping to the north." When the property owner refused to meet with a group of archaeologists who had driven up from Tennessee to study the room on Grandma's property after he had definitely agreed to meet with us, that was my first clue that attitudes had changed.

On a recent trip to Millboro, I was surprised to see that the owner of the property had erected a large mobile home directly over the larger kiva. Also, he removed all rocks and other land-marks over the smaller kiva (the one we exposed on TV) and obliterated all traces of its existence. Earlier my daughter, Evie, who regresses back to an Indian woman who lived in Robin's Nest, told me that the rooms had originally been dug by the Indians and were called "Kivas."

On a recent television show precisely geared to undermine and ridicule this work, a local (Bath County) deputy sheriff and self-appointed historian stated that the elders in the town have identi-fied these underground rooms as "cisterns." This man had earlier been an active participant in the study, even to the point of wanting me to hypnotize him.

The cistern theory holds no water whatsoever, if you will excuse the pun. Webster's dictionary describes a cistern as "a reservoir for water. A large receptacle used for storing water, usually underground." The room I looked into, and photographed, had no floor, just dirt with tree roots growing into the room. A Native American friend of mine, a member of the Vermillion tribe, explained to me that the Indians put no floor in the kivas on purpose, so that in times of heavy rain or flooding the accumulated water would simply drain off into the earth.

A few years ago, an old-timer in town was trying to convince me that the underground rooms in Millboro were part of an elaborate sewer system installed under the town. How ridiculous would it be for a town the size of Millboro to install a sewer system? I am sure there has always been an adequate system in place. In the old days they were called "out houses!"

If the people of Millboro are really interested in convincing the world that nothing unusual happened there in years past, perhaps they should just let me bring a competent team of archaeologists into town to do some carbon dating and other forms of checking—especially on the kivas.

Recently the old boarding house in Millboro was torn down. The owner told me it was necessary as the old building was succumbing to dry rot. Large slabs of concrete have been piled on top of the kiva located under the driveway that ran between the shed that stood next to the boarding house and the old bank building.

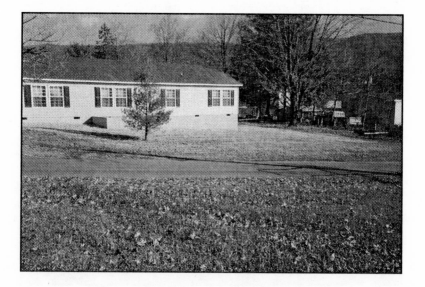

Property owner has put a mobile home over site of large kiva. Small Kiva we exposed is in front of tree at right.

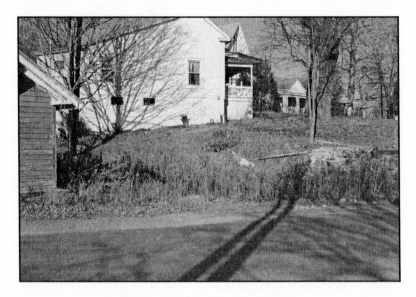

Former site of boarding house

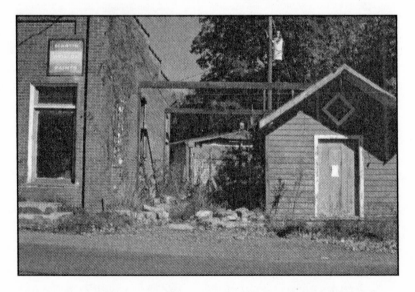

Concrete and debris piled on top of kiva under alleyway

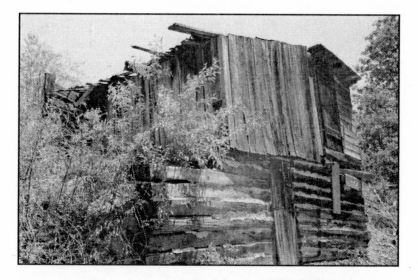

Old Confederate fort in Millboro in 1987

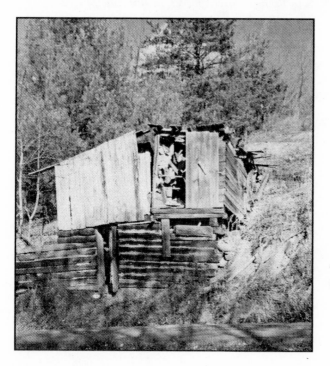

*Same fort
in 1999*

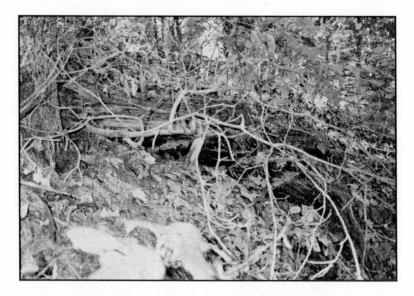

*Mouth of tunnel above church in Williamsburg
when it was first approached*

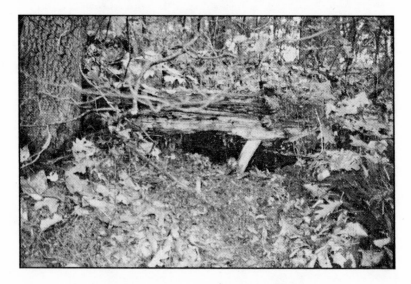

Mouth of tunnel after growth was cleared away

The old Confederate fort that stands just outside the heart of town is disintegrating at an alarming rate—a genuine piece of history left to deteriorate.

The ruins of Liz's old house that we found in 1988 were removed immediately after the publication of *Mission to Millboro*. No trace of any type remains on the property.

About half way into the research of this story, I was told by several people, mostly the ones who had lived in the Williamsville area, that the old Presbyterian Church there had a room (not a kiva, this room was built by slaves) built under the church specifically to hide escaping slaves. The church is built right into the side of a steep hill. The story was that abolitionists would drive a wagon loaded with runaway slaves, in the dead of night, across the road leading to houses directly above the church. When they reached a certain point, the wagon would stop and the slaves, following a leader, would disembark and follow the leader down the steep hillside about twenty feet or so to the opening of the tunnel, enter and crawl through the tunnel into the room under the church.

When I had my daughter Evie in Williamsville on one of our visits, she led me directly up the hill behind the church to the mouth of the tunnel, still intact. Returning later with my video and still camera, I was confronted by an irate property owner who ordered us off the property. I had been told that the church owned that property. On later visits, careful to stay on church property, I was able to get close enough to determine pretty much that the tunnel and all signs of it had been totally obliterated.

When a property owner was approached about exposing the room under her house, I was informed that her son owns the house and property and had no interest in finding the kiva.

Discourse with the owners of the Green Valley farm was equally unrewarding. I offered to go into the existing basement, carefully remove the bricks that hid the large part of the basement (where slaves and later escaping Union soldiers were hidden), take pictures of the room and tunnel leading out to Stuart Creek behind the house, and carefully reseal everything as it had been. My offer was met with an absolute, stony NO.

The Millboro residents' desire for privacy is understandable, but it does seem a shame that so much fascinating, inspiring history should be denied its place in posterity.

WARM SPRINGS INN

Directly across the highway from the old (1761) mineral bath houses in Warm Springs stands the Warm Springs Inn.

In 1790 Warm Springs was selected as the county seat of the newly formed Bath County. In the 1800s two brick buildings were erected. One housed the court house and clerk's office, the other the jail.

When the buildings were outgrown as jail and courthouse, they became the Warm Springs Inn. The large courthouse was renovated into a reception hall, bar, kitchen and spacious dining room. The jail and other out-buildings were changed into comfortable, well-appointed bedrooms.

On the porch of the old jail building, two doors are displayed. One is a large, heavy wrought iron waffle-weave door that was used to lock up a cell. The other door is a very heavy, thick wooden type that was also used to restrain prisoners.

Through the years, the prisoners did a lot of carving and engraving on the wooden door, all of which survives today. One can see a railroad locomotive, some strange animals, houses and buildings of different size and shape and many sketches of women, very naked, in sexually provocative poses. It is not difficult to discern along principally which avenue these prisoners' minds traveled.

According to the Inn's owner, a few months ago someone decided to steal the hand-carved door. They got it as far as the parking lot, but discovered it was too big and ungainly to get into their car. The owner found the door abandoned in the parking lot the next morning. Now he has the wooden door, alongside the cast-iron door, securely bolted to the porch of the old jailhouse.

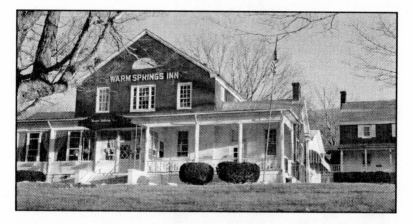

Former court house, now Warm Springs Inn

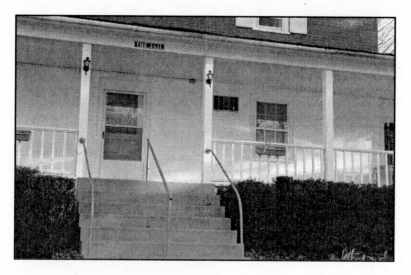

Old jail building behind former court house

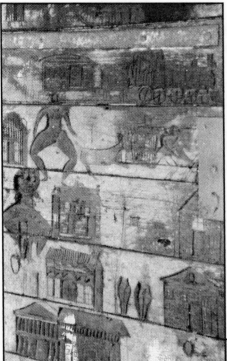

Wooden jail door hand-carved by inmates

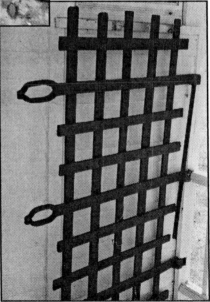

Cast-iron jail door

SUPPLIES FOR GETTYSBURG?

Recently I received a prodigious packet of maps and correspondence from Mr. Richard Borchert of Sun City Center, Florida.

Richard stated that he had avidly studied the Civil War. Because he had read that Eisenhower was chosen to be the Allied Military leader in W.W. II due to his experience in supply logistics, he realized that a great deal of any army's success depended upon a prompt and efficient supply system, including all armies in the Civil War.

For a long time Richard had been curious about the supply problems of the Civil War. He learned that Grant built a new railroad from the James River to the siege lines at Petersburg, Virginia. The operation was so extensive that a city named Hopewall grew on the James River where the line began and remains as a thriving city today.

Thanks to the Millboro story, Richard continued, he learned that Millboro was a major supply depot in the western mountains of Virginia.

On a trip to Virginia looking for Millboro, Richard and his wife became hopelessly lost, even with an up-to-date road map. "The road leading off the County road has forks and all sorts of confusing curves surrounded by thick woods with plenty of underbrush right up to within a couple of feet of the blacktop so that we didn't know where we were after leaving the main road. Our sense of direction was totally lost and the woods obscured our ability to determine the direction using the sun. Several times we ran across the railroad track that goes into Millboro, but not the town. We got very frustrated, but in the back of my mind, I kept thinking Millboro is REALLY buried back in these hills. Certainly a perfect place to hide supplies!"

Richard continued, "Your second book *(Return to Millboro)* mentioned that Samuel stole guns from the Millboro stockpile. He marveled at what beautiful rifles they were—having been made in

Belgium. To me that says they were first-class rifles, shipped all the way across the ocean, through blockades, and then transported clear across Virginia to be hidden in the mountains for clearly some very major purpose. That did a lot to reinforce my belief that the Northern invasion was that 'major purpose!'"

Richard's hypothesis is that Millboro was the major forward base to supply the Gettysburg invasion.

After months and months of intense research, necessitating trips to several out-of-the-way libraries, he has unearthed a series of Civil War railroad maps that seem to bear out his proposition. What he was looking for was a "rail system from Millboro to Gettysburg and one that was easily defended and/or concealed."

What his railroad maps reveal is that there was a "screen of mountains from Millboro to Gettysburg. The mountains screened the rail line running north from Millboro towards Gettysburg from the Shenandoah Valley proper. The screen was lost around Front Royal, Harper's Ferry and Charlestown." So while battles were fought in the Shenandoah, it was possible for the trains to sneak behind the mountain screen for the largest part of the trip to Gettysburg.

It is an established fact that some of Lee's officers and men were urging him to go hide in the mountains and continue the war guerrilla-style rather than surrender. Richard feels that that is why Lee struck out towards Appomattox when he was boxed in by Grant and forced to quit. Lee was a native of Virginia, undoubtedly very familiar with the Blue Ridge Mountains. His wife had spent a great deal of time in Warm Springs, using the warm, therapeutic spa there. To get to Warm Springs she most likely rode the train to Millboro and took a carriage on to the Springs. Probably if Lee had been able to reach supplies at Millboro he could have continued the war for an indeterminate period of time.

Richard's work shows that there clearly was a rail system connecting Millboro, Goshen, Staunton, Hagerstown and Gettysburg. He feels that there is no doubt that Lee used these railroads to

Gettysburg and probably drew supplies from Millboro principally as well as perhaps other places such as Lynchburg, but all funneling up through Staunton.

CHAPTER TWO

THE CONFEDERATE
WHITE HOUSE

DURING MY WORK WITH CHARLIE (Joe Nazarowski) while researching the Millboro story, I nurtured a nagging doubt as to why the
South would release a man as young as Charlie (22) from active
duty who had sustained fairly superficial wounds. More impor-
tantly, he was a five-year West Point graduate and a man who had
graduated extremely high in the class of 1861.

The year Joe and Maureen and I were back in Millboro, a local
Civil War buff casually remarked that it had been rumored that
Millboro had been a training ground for Confederate spies.

This remark jolted me awake to the possibility that Charlie may
have been a spy. That evening I hypnotized Joe into the role of
Charlie and asked where he had gone when his wounds healed and
if he had met with any important people. His answer was that he
was sitting around a large round table with several men. He was
wearing a dress uniform and all the other men were in uniform
except one. Then he clammed up, announcing that this was top-
secret military material that he could discuss with no one.

As Joe came out of the trance, his face had a look of total
amazement and confusion. Then he stated, "That's what changed!
I was still in uniform when I met with those men. I was never out of
the army!"

He stated that he was getting either briefed or debriefed, talking to some extremely high-ranking people. Immediately he recognized Jeb Stuart and was not certain of the other men, who all had beards except the one in civilian clothes.

The meeting was in somebody's house, around a large, very beautiful wooden table. He was being put into something called "Special Branch"—they did not call it Intelligence. The civilian present had an exceptionally cavernous face and appeared to be very important. Later he explained that it was Jefferson Davis.

Charlie was being sent as a spy to Millboro, Virginia, with a cover as a horse trainer. His orders were very specific: to secure the railroad, blow it up, also the tunnel, if the Yankees ever threatened to take Millboro.

Before the Civil War started, the Central Virginia Railroad was engaged in drilling two tunnels through two hills in downtown Millboro. This was being done so the line could be extended beyond the town, probably to Roanoke.

At the onset of the war, the first tunnel had been completed and a "turnaround" installed just beyond the tunnel. The routine went like this: A loaded freight train would pull into town and the freight cars put on sidings. Then the engine would continue on through the tunnel, slowly onto the turnaround. The engineer and other railroad men would get out and manually turn the engine around so it was facing the rear of the tunnel. Then the engine would chug back through the tunnel, pick up any empty freight cars or waiting passengers and proceed back to Staunton.

The core of Charlie's mission was to destroy that tunnel beyond repair. With the tunnel gone, the Yanks would have no way to move the supplies out of town. Charlie stated that if the supplies had fallen into Yank hands and they had moved them out of town, the war would have been over for the South in a matter of weeks.

At this meeting, he had been given a letter signed by Jefferson Davis authorizing him to seize command of the Millboro area any time he deemed it necessary and automatically promoting him to the rank of general at the same time.

Upon leaving the meeting, the civilian, whom Charlie (Joe) was now certain was Jefferson Davis, President of the Confederacy, said to him, "These are desperate and trying times. You cannot fail at this mission. It will greatly enhance our cause. Good luck and God bless you." Then they shook hands.

A few years ago there was a documentary on television about famous Southern mansions. Featured was "The Confederate White House" in Richmond, Virginia, which was Jefferson Davis' home for the duration of the war.

Obtaining a tape of this documentary, I prepared to show it to Joe, in the role of Charlie, to see if he recognized any part of the old house.

First, I got him to relate the story in more detail. As soon as he was discharged from the hospital, some men came and got him. He does not know who they were, but they had authorization papers ordering him to Richmond. They took him to Richmond in a carriage in which the windows were covered. It was hot and dusty so we can assume it was summer. The air was close in the carriage but they would not let him uncover the windows. (Obviously they did not want him to be seen by anyone who might recognize him. Official military records of the time list Charles Patterson as dying from wounds a few days after the battle of Shiloh.)

The trip took about two days, and upon arrival at Richmond he was taken somewhere where he could clean up prior to the meeting with the President. He left for the meeting in full dress uniform.

His escorts to the Presidential home were the same men who had picked him up at the hospital. He was told neither where he was going or with whom he would be meeting.

Charlie did not enter the house through the front door. In fact, according to him, he did not even *see* the front door. His carriage went around to the side of the house and parked.

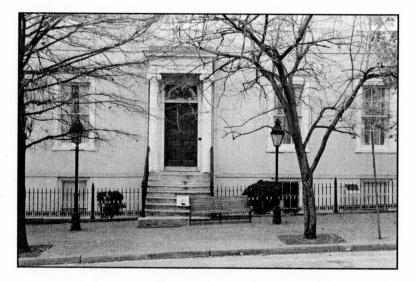

Front door, Confederate White House

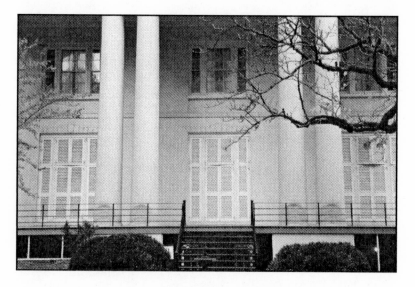

Rear door and porch of White House

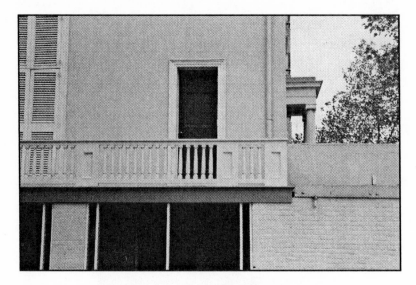

Side door used by Charlier Patterson
to enter and leave White House

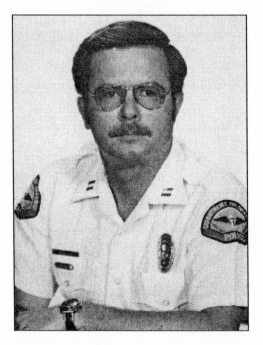

Joe Nazarowski,
whose alter ego
in the Millboro
story was
"Chalie Patterson"

At this juncture, I asked if it was an office building of some type. "No, it is an old house. A very big house." Continuing, he explained that he did not see any part of the house except that one side (a side, incidentally, that was and is well hidden from prying eyes in the area, especially from the street).

There were a couple of men waiting for him as he went up the steps, and they escorted him into the house through the side door. They walked down a short hall, then through another side door into a large room. "I would say it was a dining room; it's too big to be a parlor."

The table he was so taken with was about eight feet across, four feet deep, oblong in shape. Originally he had stated it was oak, but now he was not certain of the wood. It was, however, very hard wood and very impressive.

Then he stated emphatically, "Nice chairs!" The furniture in the room was all large, ornate and carved. He was also impressed by a large piece of furniture along the wall, probably a serving sideboard. "Very elegant!"

Inquiring, I asked if the floor was hardwood and bare. "No, it's covered by a rose-colored carpet, pinkish red color, gorgeous!"

When it was suggested that he glance into the other rooms, he answered, "There are a couple of doors leading out of the room, but they are closed. I cannot see into any other rooms."

Again he identified one of the military men as Jeb Stuart and was unsure of the identity of any of the others, but he was more certain that the civilian was Jeff Davis.

Then he viewed the videotape of the Confederate White House. Immediately, when it came on the screen, he identified the side door through which he had entered. He did not recognize the front of the house or the back, overlooking the beautiful flower garden.

He became alert when the large room came on the screen, exclaiming once again about the exquisite carpeting. When the large oval table appeared, he became very excited and identified it as the one at which he had sat. Later a chandelier was shown, but he denied that he had seen it, declaring, "The chandelier I saw was more ornate." Noting a picture of George Washington on the wall, he denied it was there when he visited the room in 1862.

The group instructed him to wear knockabout clothes from this point on and to hide his uniform. As an aside, he declared that he was still in a state of shock that such high-ranking people were interested in conferring with him. When asked what rank he was, he answered, "Captain." Learning that the record listed him as a Lt. Colonel, he replied, "My permanent rank was that of Captain. I was breveted, temporarily promoted to Lt. Colonel."

Declaring that they gave him five days to get things in order, he again quoted what Davis had said to him about the importance of blowing up the tunnel.

Recently I had a chance to visit the Confederate White House in Richmond, Virginia. The tour proved that everything Joe had said, in trance, was absolutely true. The large oval table is situated in what had been the dining room. The carpet was exactly as he had described it. Unfortunately the guide forbade picture-taking inside the house, but I was able to get shots of the exterior. At the end of the tour, we left the dining room and walked down the short hallway that ran along the dining room and exited through the side door, exactly as Charlie Patterson had.

An interesting note. The front door of the house is directly on the street, as houses were built in that era. No front yard, no walkway. The front is extremely plain. The guide explained that in those days, all garbage and refuse was thrown out in the street, and little attention was paid to the front of the house. On the other hand, the rear of the dwelling is spectacular. A huge veranda, or porch, runs the entire width of the house, with large, white antebellum columns extending to the ceiling. The veranda overlooks a delightful, large garden with winding paths running through it.

CHAPTER THREE

MILLBORO

WHILE JOE, MAUREEN AND I were on a flight to Washington, D.C., to appear on the *Larry King Show* (shortly after *Mission to Millboro* had been released), I glanced at Maureen, sitting between myself and Joe, Her white-knuckled hands were clenching either arm rest and her face was ashen. Maureen is terrified to fly, and I had forgotten this fact.

On an earlier trip east, I had had to hypnotize her to get her onto the airplane. Of course I had forgotten what I had said previously to get her on board, but one look told me I had better think of something, pronto!

Taking her hand in mine, I counted her into a trance. She immediately became limp and relaxed. Now, I wondered, how do I keep her this way? There was absolutely no time for lengthy anti-flight-fear lessons. After giving some reassuring suggestions, I stated that I would count her awake on the count of five.

"But now," I continued, "I will count to four, and part of your mind will awaken. The part that is causing you to be afraid will remain asleep. And it will remain asleep until I say five."

Then I proceeded to count to four, and Mo opened her eyes and immediately began an animated conversation with Joe.

After landing at Dulles Airport, I took Mo aside, put my hand on her shoulder, snapped my fingers, and said, "Five." She shook her head and announced, "Now I am wide awake."

This same wile worked equally as well when I had Lynn and Evie (Martha and Roy, both characters in *Return to Millboro)* back in Millboro and about to cross the Cowpasture River on a steel suspension bridge. Both girls took one look at the bridge and announced firmly that they were never, no way, going to walk across it. It was scary, about eighty feet above the river which was full of huge, sharp rocks and broiling, churning water. A prevailing breeze would cause the bridge to sway eerily.

I hypnotized the two of them, gave them the same suggestions I had given Maureen on the plane, and soon they were trotting cheerfully behind me on the bridge. As the bridge swayed in an uncanny motion, I could hear them behind me saying, "Whee!"

On the trip back I used the same tactic and, after regaining solid ground, my daughter looked at me and proclaimed, "Mother, I can't believe you got me to walk across that silly bridge, not once but twice!"

Probably the most excitement I experienced while researching the Millboro story is when I went back to the town with a TV producer, and we exposed an underground room which one of my characters had told me about.

The character was Sally (Lenette Brychel). She was a young girl who had lived in Millboro with her grandma while the story was unfolding. At the end of the regression, while still hypnotized, she casually mentioned that in Grandma's house, if you rolled up the rug in the dining room, there was a trap door in front of the fireplace that led to an underground room where Grandma hid escaping slaves.

When she awakened from the trance, I handed her a large picture of the old town taken shortly after the Civil War that a deputy sheriff had given me several years earlier. When asked if she could see Grandma's house in the picture, she said she could. I handed her a pen, and she made a large "X" on the house.

After several letters and phone calls, I located the owner of the property. (The house had burned down a year or two earlier.) He

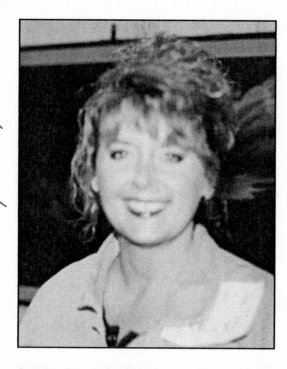

*Lenette Brychel marked an "X" on a picture
of Grandma's house*

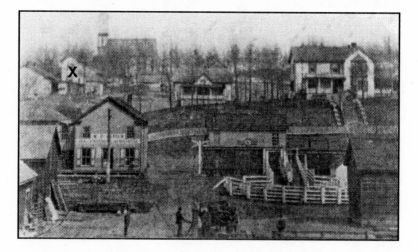

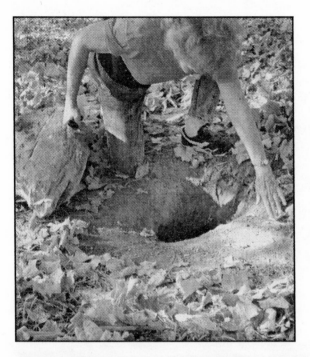

*Author peers
down into
underground
room on
"Grandma's"
property.*

Photo by
Bob Smith
of the Cayce
Foundation

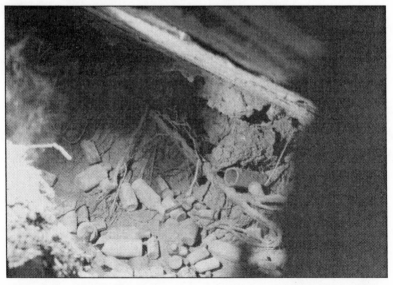

Underground room under Grandma's house

was excited and told me that when he tore down the old shed on the property, he had unearthed a large hole that had to lead to either a tunnel or room below.

Sally had said that there were two rooms. The one under the house was largest; that's where the slaves ate and slept. Then there was a tunnel about four or five feet long that ran into a smaller room that led up into the shed—this was where they brought the slaves out in the dead of night.

Prior to leaving to go back East, I had called Lenette and hypnotized her over the phone. When directed to describe the underground room, she said, "It's about the size of a small, one-car garage. The other room is larger. It has ugly, bilious green-colored walls, and the ceiling is rough-hewn wood. The floor is dirt, like a mine shaft, and now there are roots growing into it." When we got back to Millboro, the property owner had dug, with his backhoe, a tunnel about four feet deep alongside the room. Then he broke a hole into the wall of the room the size of a pie pan.

No one can imagine my reaction when I crawled down into that trench and shone my one-half-million-candlepower lamp into the room. The first thing my eyes met was the bilious green wall. My daughter Evie had told me Indians built this and the other rooms around Millboro. They are called kivas. The walls are green, she said, because the Indians mixed the concrete with local sulfur water, which later turned the mixture green.

Then, with the hair on the back of my head standing at attention, I shone the light upwards. There I saw the rough-hewn wooden ceiling. Evie said the Indians felled the trees and planed the wood. They did all this, including digging the rooms, using only rocks and bones as tools. This was one of the most exciting moments of my life!

When *Mission to Millboro* was first published, the people in the town were, of course, excited. Immediately some of the old-timers picked up on a glaring error in the book. When Maureen and Joe and I were back there, she took a picture of an old shed located below the old Confederate fort. Later she informed me that this shed was where Samuel and John used to meet, and I said so in the book.

Later, when Mo and Smokey and I were in Millboro together, they pointed out an old shed behind (and much nearer) to the fort and stated that that shed was where the meetings were held. Since the first shed named was built around W.W. II, of course, it was not there during the Civil War. When I asked Maureen why she had made the statement about the first shed, she simply admitted, "I made a mistake!"

This mistake appears to have turned a lot of the townspeople against this story, and many of them now believe the whole tale is contrived and made up. This is most unfortunate. Everything I write is what I learn from these people while in trance. It would take a much better writer than myself to dream up a story of this scope and magnitude. After the *Sightings* show on Fox TV aired, showing pictures of the underground room, the town immediately shut down (to me, that is).

It had been arranged for us to meet with several archaeologists from Tennessee. They drove up to Millboro to meet us. However, the owner of the site of Grandma's house failed to keep the appointment, after saying he would.

When I requested permission to go into the main basement of the Green Valley farm and photograph the area where the slaves were hidden, it was flatly denied. The Presbyterian Church in Williamsville vehemently denied me permission to expose the hidden room under the church. When I pointed out a small air pipe leading to the room on the church yard, it was removed. When my daughter led me up the steep hill behind the church and showed me the opening of the tunnel the slaves had used to enter the hidden room, the property owner appeared. I had thought we were on church property but such was not the case. The land owner threatened to have us arrested, put in jail and possibly shot for trespassing.

After giving me written permission to dig anywhere I chose on his property, the owner of the old boarding house parked his pickup truck directly over the kiva, preventing me from exposing it.

The owners of the lot next to the fire station (where a big kiva is located) refused even to speak to me. The owner of the Cauthorn house "had no interest" in exposing the room on his property.

Even up in Robin's Nest, the neat rows of crops, which had been reseeding since the Indians were chased out after the Civil War, were, at my last visit, all obliterated.

I can sympathize with the townpeople's concern for their privacy, but what a shame that history is being denied knowledge of these fascinating artifacts.

There were several people who were in the Millboro study who, for one reason or another, failed to make it into the book.

One was Rose, the woman who ran the bawdy house in Millboro during the Civil War and was a Union spy and a compadre of John's. She, today, is a very elderly woman who lives in Lake Elsinore. She, as with most of the others, looks today a great deal as Rose did in the 1800s. She is dark-haired, fair-skinned, with lovely gray eyes and remnants of a gorgeous body.

Rose tells of renting the whorehouse from one of the men in town. He was an extremely unpleasant man who constantly berated her for what she was doing, while chasing after the girls all the time he was there. She thought that it was a good chance that he was Constance's father.

She recognized pictures of all the people in the town, especially Ruthie (who had come to work in her house). She was familiar with the old man who had abused Ruthie, and said he came to the house and caused a lot of trouble, trying to get her back. Looking at a picture of John, she claimed he was a good friend; he came to the house a lot. She admitted there was "some sort of intrigue" with John. They were both Union spies who collaborated, which she eventually admitted.

Rose's real name was Rosemary. She was a widow with three children who were all grown when the war started. She was approached by the Union to go to Millboro and open the house and spy. She did not ever feel right about what she was doing— operating the house, that is.

Rose was especially careful that her children not know what she was doing. The up-side was that she made a great deal of money, both with the house and the bar. Rose did not feel as though her life had been a happy one.

Another character is a woman who currently lives in Canyon Lake, an area very near Lake Elsinore. She gave the name of Anna. Anna Kent. Anna was an Indian girl, about sixteen when we talked to her.

She was an infant when Union troops raided her village. Both her parents were killed, and one of the soldiers picked up the terrified, crying little baby and took her home to his wife. There were two older children, and Anna was accepted into the family.

When her step-father was released from the Army, they moved to Millboro Springs onto a farm. Eventually two other children were born. Anna did not look at all like an Indian and was raised as a white girl, attending school with her four siblings.

Her life was normal until she grew up. She socialized and was accepted as were her brothers and sisters. However, her parents knew full well she was Indian, so she was never allowed a relationship with a man.

The other children married and left, but Anna remained home with her step-parents. When they died, she stayed on in the farm house until her own death in her late thirties.

Anna's story, like John's, exemplifies the tragedy of the racism of the time. She was neither fish nor fowl. Raised as a white girl, she was allowed all the advantages of the white race except being allowed to marry and fulfill her life. That she was Indian was never discussed. She had no opportunity to ever meet or cultivate a friendship with her own race. She was totally segregated from them, not that they would have accepted her after being raised among "the enemy." How many lives were ruined in this way we certainly never will know.

In the book *Return to Millboro,* I mention a prominent movie star who is, unbeknownst to himself, a part of the story.

I will refer to him as "Fred Jones."

One day Maureen said to me, "I see Fred Jones, the movie star, back there in Millboro." Fascinated, I asked what she saw him doing. "I dunno," she answered, "I just see him back there." Later I asked Evie if she saw Fred Jones in Millboro (she was in a trance at the time). Immediately she responded that, yes, she saw him. He was the blacksmith she claimed. Further, she stated that one or more of Fred's children were there also.

Later I discussed this with Maureen and she retorted, "Ask Joe. I see him in the saloon drinking with Charlie."

Next time Joe was at my house, I hypnotized him back into the role of Charlie and inquired about Fred Jones. Thoughtfully he answered, "Yes, that could be him—by golly, it is him." I inquired what he was doing. Charlie answered, "I see him pounding an anvil." Playing dumb I inquired what an anvil was. "He's the blacksmith; he's shoeing a horse." Later he stated that they were good friends, drank together nightly in the saloon. Occasionally he would go with Fred and help him salvage railroad tracks that the Yanks had torn up. This was his only source of metal with which to shoe the horses.

Another time Becky (Maureen) said that she saw him in a funny-looking uniform. He was in the "Home Guard," synonymous with our National Guard today. Among the many things he did in the Home Guard was to help run the Indians out of Robin's Nest.

The interesting upshot of this story is that in this life "Fred Jones" is very much a political activist and a staunch supporter of Indian causes. Perhaps this is an indication of how "karma" works.

CHAPTER FOUR

THE BIG WHITE ROCK

BECAUSE I AM DEFINITELY PERSONNA NON GRATA in the town of Millboro, I set my sights on Robin's Nest, high on a mountaintop above the town. Robin's Nest is located in the George Washington National Forest and open to everyone, especially a taxpayer like myself.

I decided to search out the big white rock of which I have heard so much. Almost everyone affiliated with the story, at one time or another, mentions the big white rock, especially the Indians. To them it was a big-time religious icon.

A couple of years ago, I thought we had found it. Several persons in town said if I took the highway out of Goshen and looked up, I would see it. Well, I did. There at the top of the three-thousand-foot Mill Mountain resides a large out cropping of white quartz which I immediately assumed was our rock. It was not, but I did not know that at the time.

An acquaintance of mine arranged for us to go up to a hunting lodge at the top of a nearby mountain. From there we could hike across the crest of the mountains to Mill Mountain and to the rock. Sometimes we walked on ground that was no more than two feet wide, a three-thousand-foot straight down drop on either side. Sometimes we crawled on all fours over sharp, pointed rocks, but we finally got to the gray rock, above the white quartz. By then it was late, and we had to head back. Immediately it started to rain.

Not a gentle, soft rain. More like a driving, blinding downpour, drenching us to the skin and making it impossible to see, especially if one had glasses on.

Somehow we made it back to the car.

The next fall we returned: Joann Kelly (Soaring Eagle), who, as S.E., had told me much about the rock; Steve, a young TV producer from Georgia who had driven up from Atlanta to meet us; and Ron, a friend of mine.

In good spirits we all set out. After all, we knew where we were headed. We drove to the hunting lodge and started out across the crest of the mountains. The last thing the owner of the lodge had said to us the year before was, "Stay on the crest, and you will be okay. Stray down the mountainside and you will get into trouble."

Those words should be cast in concrete and mounted on the top of every mountain in the area. Off we started, fat, dumb and happy. We all had sandwiches in our backpacks, and Ron was carrying the water for all of us, something he insisted was a good idea.

It was difficult to stay on the crest of the mountain. In some areas the crest widens out, and one is not sure where the crest is. You find yourself walking along the side of the mountain.

On one such wide area, I changed my course and headed back for the crest, assuming the rest would follow. We were near the gray rock, and I was anxious to reach that point so we could go down the mountain one hundred feet or so to the white rock.

I was chugging along, looking to neither right or left, when Steve joined me. "Where are the others?" I asked. "Oh," he retorted, "they decided to go another route."

It was difficult for me to believe what I was hearing. One of the Cardinal rules of an expedition of this type is to STAY TO-GETHER! To separate is disaster, as everyone discovered later that day.

Steve and I reached the gray rock. He stopped to eat a sandwich. I could not eat because my mouth was very dry, and RON HAD ALL THE WATER!

After Steve ate, we started slowly down the mountain beside the gray rock.

My theory was that Joann and Ron had decided to cut across the side of the mountain to the white rock. If this was the case and they were successful (which I seriously doubted), then we would intersect them somewhere down by the white rock.

Steve and I were down the mountain about forty feet when the going got rougher and rougher, the slope got steeper and steeper. I suggested that we try to get back up to the crest, and he said that would be almost impossible. Looking back, I realize we should have gone for it; it couldn't have been as bad as what we faced all afternoon.

Unwisely, I said, "Okay, we'll walk down the mountain." Walk? I don't think so! We ended up sliding on our butts. We would let go of one tree and slide, rapidly, and crash into another tree. As we were sliding down Mill Mountain, I hurriedly pointed out the white rock on our left to Steve. Finally the trees gave out to

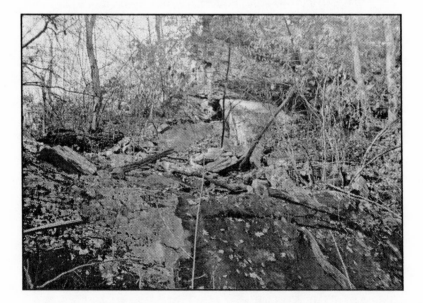

Crest of mountain was almost impassable

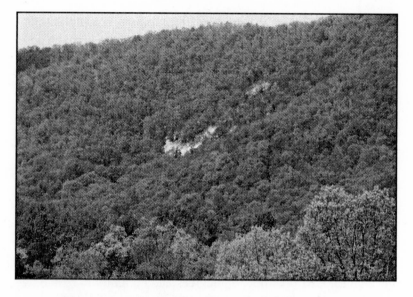

The wrong white rock at the top of Mill Mountain

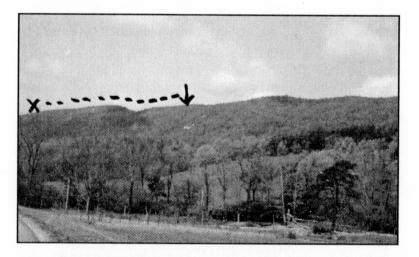

"X" marks the hunting lodge. Arrow shows location of rock. Broken lines show distance hiked.

thick underbrush. And I mean THICK! Walking was nigh impossible, but we made it through somehow. There was so much dead brush that every step was a hazard. About every other step your foot would drop down into a deep, hidden hole. How we ever made it down without breaking a leg, I'll never know.

After about two and one-half hours of slogging through the impenetrable underbrush and fighting the thorny vines, we made it to a logging road. My left arm was bleeding so badly I had to remove my watch so it wouldn't get ruined.

Aha! I thought, seeing the logging road. "We're saved." Not to be. We were hopelessly lost. We could hear the traffic on the highway, but where was it? In which direction? We spent another two or three hours hopelessly following logging roads.

At one juncture we passed a turkey farm. At least that is what the sign said. Bt this time, 98 degrees and humidity to match, we were both seriously dehydrated. Steve went to search for water, and I admonished him, "I don't care if you have to wrestle all the turkeys to the ground, GET THEIR WATER!"

Unfortunately everything was locked up tight, and there was no water anywhere.

We struggled along, and eventually I became convinced that the traffic was closer. At my insistence, we struck off through more high, thick underbrush and close trees and eventually came within sight of the highway. We located a chicken farm, and a lovely young lady who gave us gallons of pineapple juice and water. Then she graciously drove us home.

An hour or two later, Joann and Ron staggered in. They had regained the crest, come to the gray rock, started down, fought their way back up, walked back to the car, and spent a couple of hours driving around in the car looking for us. Their intentions were good, but believe me, no car ever went where Steve and I had been!

Many times while researching the Millboro story, I have been diverted onto a wild goose chase. We spent days trying to ascertain which was the Cauthorn house. There is another, badly run-down house close into town which we were convinced was the house we were after. It was when I had Pat Greene (John in the Millboro story) in Millboro that he led me to the Cauthorn house, stating it was the one to which he had seen escaping slaves run.

Another time, Smokey and I were searching desperately for Bratton's Bridge. We had driven over it several times, but Smokey said, no, there were two sets of railroad tracks when he and John led the Yank soldiers out from under the bridge. Finally, he talked to a store owner near Goshen, and the owner explained there used to be a railroad spur running onto the Bratton property. The spur was removed around the time of World War II. This was later confirmed to me by a member of the Bratton family.

When Joann Kelley and I were looking desperately for the white rock, an acquaintance of mine in Millboro said it was high up on the side of Mill Mountain towards Goshen. When we looked up and saw it, we figured that it had to be the Indian's white rock.

However, as we slid down the mountain past the rock, I realized that that could not be the rock for which we searched. The Indian's rock was a serious religious icon, in front of which they held religious ceremonies. Several of the Indians in the Millboro study said they used to play around the bottom of the rock and try to climb it when they were children. I can guarantee you that, even if through some miracle children could get near that rock we visited, no children could ever play there.

The reason I am searching so assiduously for the Indian's white rock is because, for the past couple of years, two of the Indians, Running Springs (Evie) and Soaring Eagle (Joann) have regaled me with tales of a cave near the rock. The cave has petroglyphs on the walls and a large painting of some sort on the ceiling.

Beyond the cave, and connected to it, is a large cavernous area which contains more pictures. I directed Joann, while in the role of Soaring Eagle, to draw a sketch of the petroglyphs, and he drew the usual sun, animal, rain and flowing water. Then he drew ⚬⚬. When I asked what that sign meant, he stated, "Our paths will

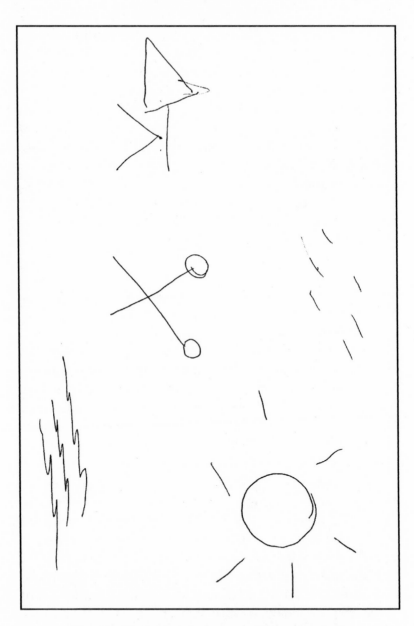

*Soaring Eagle sketched some of the petroglyphs
that are in the cave*

cross." Later, when I hypnotized Evie and asked Springs what the symbol meant, I heard, "We will meet again."

The cavern beyond the cave winds on endlessly, and they both warned me not to go too far into it as I could easily get lost. It seems that several Indians, at various times got into the cavern, became lost and perished. Eagle became very emotional one time when he was talking about this. Suddenly he started to cry, then he explained, "I see the body of a very young boy. He got into the cavern and could not find his way out. He died, there in the cave. He was my younger brother. We always assumed he had been killed by a bear.

Several corridors led off from the main cavern, and there are very small rooms (sealed up) that are tombs, tombs that contain very ancient bodies. Also many Indian artifacts are to be found in the cave. According to Running Springs the arrow that Eagle used to kill the deer during his "manhood ritual" is ensconced in the cave.

By searching and talking to some of the few friendly locals, I was able to locate another white rock. Much smaller than the first one, it is equally inaccessible but much closer to Robin's Nest.

Talking to Running Springs one day prior to a trip back to Millboro, she discussed the rock. "I see it now; it does not stand out as it usually does. It has green grass growing all over it. Covered with green grass!" This seemed very strange to me. We all know that grass does not grown on a rock. While my friend was discussing the smaller rock, she said, "It is now pretty much covered with lichen." I snapped to attention upon hearing this. What Springs was seeing was not grass but green lichen.

My first trip to the rock was with Joann Kelley and a young girl named Sharon who was interested in videotaping the expedition. As I was winded from the long trek up the trail, I remained above while the girls went searching. Eagle (Joann) had previously told me that the entrance to the cave was on the left side of the rock as one looks at it from the front of the rock. Consequently it would be on the right side as one looks at the rock from the trail. The girls started down the right side, were not gone too long and returned on the left side. They were excited. They had found something. Sharon announced, "There's a stream running into it." Hearing this I forgot about being tired. Several times when discussing the rock, Springs had stated firmly, "There's a stream running into it."

The next day we all made our way down the tortuous mountainside. We went down the right side despite the fact that the girls had stated the other side of the rock was much easier to travel. I was behind Sharon, and when I tried to get up on a flat rock, I grabbed a small tree. The tree was dead and broke off in my hand. Falling backward down the rock, I somersaulted down into a small, rock-filled pool below, landing on my head after an eight to ten-foot fall.

Badly bruised and bleeding profusely, the girls managed to pull me from the pool. Then, despite the blood running into my eyes, I was able to crawl on my hands and knees up the three hundred feet of steep mountainside to the trail.

Descending the trail at a pretty fast clip, we made it back to the car. After a forty-five-minute drive back to Hot Springs, I ended up in the emergency room of the local hospital where it took nineteen stitches to close my gaping wounds. That ended that trip. It was several weeks later when I recalled Springs telling me, "You will fall over backward, and your head will be right next to the cave opening."

Feeling sorry for me and knowing how disappointed I was, Ron (who by now was my husband) took me back to Virginia the next month to scope out the potential cave opening, after my stitches were removed.

Carefully we wended our way down the mountainside, hanging onto clothesline rope which we secured to a tree at the top of the mountain. When we reached the area where I had fallen, I looked carefully, and there, exactly where Soaring Eagle had said it was, I spotted the opening to the cave. The stream that ran alongside the "table rock" from which I had fallen divided just beyond the rock

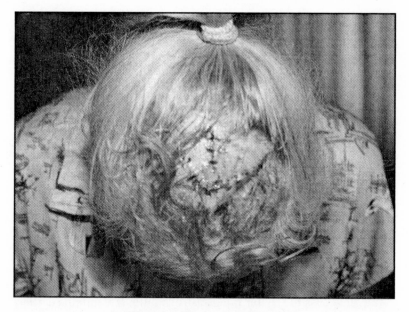

Author's head after mountain fall

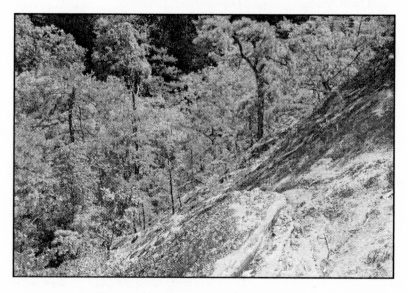

White rock extends down mountainside

and a small segment, about seven inches wide, ran directly into an opening in the rock. It had to be the cave entrance. Because we had no tools other than our hands, we decided to come back the following spring in an attempt to enter the cave. The opening in the rock was quite small, but we decided that if we dug down a ways into the soft dirt, away from the flowing stream of water, we could gain access to the cave.

The following May we returned. What a shock! We discovered in the area where I had fallen, the rocks had shifted radically. The entire mountainside was changed and distorted. The pool into which I had fallen was torn all apart and about twelve feet further down the stream. Rocks were scattered wildly about, and there was water everywhere. It looked as if some mythical giant had taken a huge mallet and smashed the entire area. Further down, the opening in the rocks was still there but much smaller, harder to see and totally inaccessible. After my disastrous fall a few months earlier, we decided not to attempt entering the cave.

Upon returning home, I hypnotized Evie and talked to Running Springs. She said there had been a series of earth movements of small earthquakes that had rearranged things down the mountainside. At that time she also made an interesting observation. "The part of the mind that survives death becomes part of a larger whole [Carl Jung's theory of the collective unconscious?] and each time one contacts it, it becomes more difficult to disengage itself from the whole.

Each time I was down the mountainside, I was overwhelmed with a deep sense of foreboding—as though an unseen presence was there, warning us to stay away. While I was down by the cave opening, all I wanted to do was flee. The feeling stayed with me until I regained solid ground at the top of the mountain.

Further discussing the cave with Springs, she stated, "When you walk into the cave, you don't go straight ahead, you go down, like a hillside." I had an inspiration and asked if it was really a cave or a cavern. She stated, "It's a cavern, a very large cavern. There's

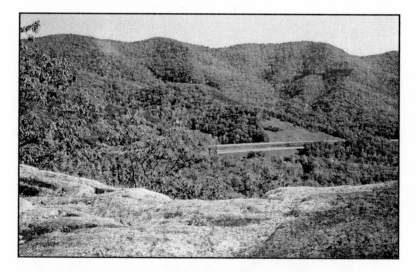

The "Overlook" provides a nice view of the valley.

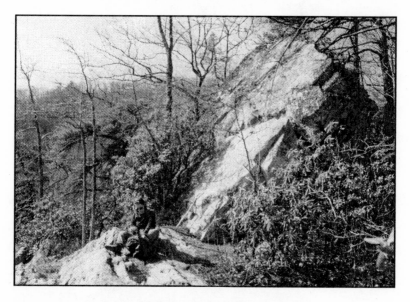

Joann Kelly rests near the overlook.
The top of the white rock is behind her.
Photo by Steve Sakalarius

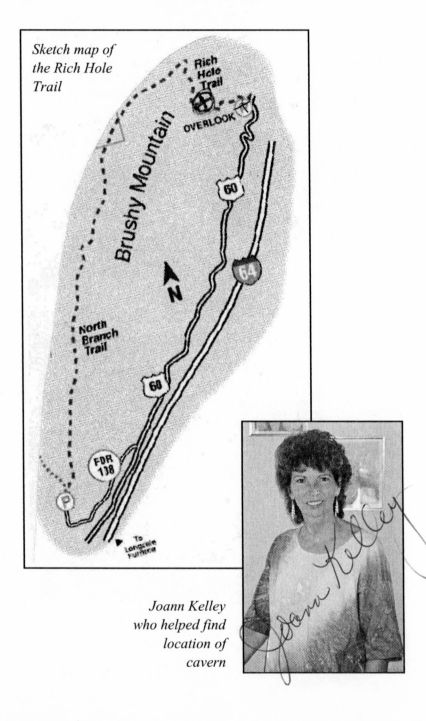

Sketch map of
the Rich Hole
Trail

*Joann Kelley
who helped find
location of
cavern*

a lake in it, and I see stalactites and stalagmites." This surprised me and later I quizzed Eagle about it and heard, "All I could see was many corridors leading off the main room. Many people got lost down there."

Years ago, when the Indians were living in Robin's Nest, the area in front of the rock was kept cleared off by the natives. According to what they tell me, it was about one half the size of a football field. There were many ceremonies held there, and it was used by all the tribes in the area. Springs once said, "The white rock was our gift from God." Some believed the rock contained healing powers and healing ceremonies were conducted in the clearing in front of the rock. Since the Indians were run out of the area, probably shortly after the Civil War, the forest has regained the land.

According to the Indians, there were and are other entrances into and out of the cavern. Eagle told of one time when he bravely decided to investigate the area in its entirely. He walked for a very long time and finally exited through an opening on the mountain-side. Admitting that he had become very frightened half-way through the trek, he stated that he was overwhelmed with relief when he finally found his way out.

On my last trip to the rock, I was accompanied by Joann Kelley and a video producer named Steve, the same Steve with whom I trudged down the side of Mill Mountain one warm, humid, water-less afternoon. When we arrived at the area where the cave entrance had been, we discovered that the same mythical giant who had created so much havoc a year earlier had really done a job this time! The huge table rock was completely gone, as was the stream. They have been replaced by countless huge, multi-ton boulders every-where. The water is still there, but instead of a stream, it bubbles up in small pools around the rocks. Standing close to the white rock, I could hear the unmistakable sound of a viable, fast-moving water-fall ... INSIDE THE ROCK! There was our cavern.

After sustaining numerous cuts, contusions, bruises, dislo-cated knees and nineteen stitches on my scalp, the realization has finally dawned on me! Perhaps it's going to take professional people who know what they are doing.

Archaeologists have tools such as resistivity meters and magnetometers to help locate anomalies under the ground. A resistivity meter is used by passing electric current between metal probes pushed into the earth. A magnetometer detects differences in the magnetic field of the soil. These devices have been around for a while. Newer techniques such as echo-sounding and soil scanning radar are more recent. (Source: *An Introduction to Archaeology,* Leslie & Roy Adkins, Shooting Star Press, N.Y., N.Y.)

One point cannot be emphasized too strongly. Bear in mind that this area is a National Forest, and only preliminary searches may be made. Any extensive digging, etc., must be discussed with the local forest rangers and proper permits obtained.

The "Big White Rock," which we finally determined to be the one we sought, is at the north end of the Rich Hole walking trail, located in the Rich Hole Wilderness. Rich Hole was thusly named because of the deep, nutritiously organic soils that constitute the area. There is an overlook area at the very north end of the trail; the overlook is adjacent to the white rock. The view from the overlook is fantastic and looks down upon Highway 64, off in the distance.

Approximately six miles in length, the trail passes through the southern half of the wilderness. The closest towns of any size are Lexington, about twelve miles away, Goshen, approximately ten miles to the north, and Clifton Forge, nine miles west.

CHAPTER FIVE

HYPNOSIS

THERE ARE AS MANY DEFINITIONS OF HYPNOSIS as there are persons practicing it. The most generally accepted one is "an altered state of consciousness," which is accurate but broad.

No one really knows exactly what happens to cause a person to become hypnotized. What appears to transpire is that the conscious mind, or critical sensor, is repressed and, to varying degrees, deactivated. This renders the emotional, unconscious part of the mind unable to reason or distinguish reality from unreality and hence extremely vulnerable to suggestion.

Many persons have made the statement, "I cannot be hypnotized; I am too strong-willed." Neither of these points are correct. Will power has absolutely nothing to do with a person's hypnotizability, nor does his level of intelligence, with the exception of the mentally retarded who have trouble sustaining concentration.

Hypnosis appears to be a delicate interworking between the body and mind which is much more a physical, or possibly genetic, action than most people realize.

Hypnosis has been compared, in a way, to electricity. Both are a powerful force that cannot be seen but are definitely felt under certain conditions. Each, when properly harnessed and directed, can contribute greatly to our lives.

The average person harbors groundless fears regarding hypnosis, the forerunner being, "Suppose you cannot bring me out of it?"

Believe me, it is much easier to bring a person out of a trance than to get them into one. If a hypnotized person were to be abandoned by the hypnotist, he would stay in the trance for an indeterminate length of time—depending on the depth of trance and the person's susceptibility to hypnosis. After a while his trance state would convert to a condition of normal sleep and after a few more minutes, he would calmly awaken.

There are instances of a person afflicted with multiple person-alities presenting problems to a hypnotist. This is an excellent example of why it is important that a person desiring to become a hypnotist get adequate training before undertaking the venture. There are some persons it is better not to hypnotize—those with a record of mental illness or those who appear to be highly unstable. It is a frightening experience for an untrained hypnotist to have a subject experience an emotion-charged, violent abreaction while in a trance. That hypnotist had better know how to handle the situa-tion, or he may end up a lot more upset than his subject. Unless the goal of the hypnotic session is emotional catharsis, the highly charged situations are best avoided.

As far as any permanent, serious mental side effects resulting from hypnosis, there is nothing to fear. Dr. William Kroger, a prominent Los Angeles psychiatrist (who has been dubbed "the father of modern hypnosis") has stated, "It is safe to say that hypnosis is the safest of all psychotherapies. Deaths and consider-able permanent damage have been reported with shock therapy, steroid administration, narcosynthesis and hallucinogenic agents. Yet no one has ever died from hypnosis." *(Clinical and Experimen-tal Hypnosis,* William Kroger, M.D., J.B. Lippencott Co., Philadel-phia). It is my personal opinion that hypnosis will not precipitate a psychotic break nor will it exacerbate any existing mental condi-tion.

It is also my opinion that one's ability to enter the hypnotic trance is predetermined in the genetic background of that person. Some people are able to become hypnotized very easily in a matter of minutes, while others require many hours of hard work and concentration. It has, however, been my experience that no one is immune from or incapable of becoming hypnotized if they are willing to devote enough time and effort to the process except, as previously mentioned, those persons who lack the mental development to sustain concentration.

Learning to become hypnotized is comparable to learning to walk. Some babies are able to stand and walk independently as early as seven or eight months. Others crawl for a while, hang on to anything available, fall down a lot, and eventually are able to maneuver by themselves as late as two years of age. The point here is that unless physically handicapped, every person does eventually, in his own time and fashion, learn to walk upright. The same principle holds for hypnosis—everyone can learn it.

The only thing predictable about hypnosis is its total unpredictability. This is why Sigmund Freud abandoned it. He thought he had discovered the perfect pathway to the unconscious mind until he experienced several failures. It has been said that Freud was unwilling to devote himself to mastering proper hypnotic procedures. From what we know of the man, it is reasonable to assume that he would discard anything that challenged his authoritarian image. One thing is certain, that there is nothing more challenging (or deflating) than a subject who refuses to become hypnotized despite the ploys of the hypnotist. Time and prolonged effort are the only factors that will eventually overcome this resistance (which again, is not necessarily only in the mind). Freud was either unaware that time could solve this problem, or he was too impatient and busy to expend the time.

Contrary to popular belief, hypnosis is not a truth serum. If a person is prone to lie in the conscious state, he will not hesitate to do so when hypnotized. Should he become annoyed or frustrated with the hypnotist, he is capable of manufacturing weird, lurid tales should he so desire. The unconscious mind, at times, appears to be totally autonomous and divorced from the conscious mind.

This fact was portrayed very clearly to me several years ago when I conducted my first serious hypnotic regression. The subject was a young woman thirty-seven years old. When regressed into a "past life' area, she described the life of a woman who was a queen in a Scandinavian country many years past. Giving the name of Priscilla, she described the woman's life in colorful, if convoluted, detail. A few months later, it was discovered that she had been reliving the life of a Swedish queen named Christina. It was an astute Swedish historian who noted that she had Anglicized the name Christina into Priscilla: they both mean pure or chaste, both have nine letters, and both contain a "ris" sound. This says something for the independent reasoning power of the unconscious mind.

It is a popular misconception that a hypnotized person can be made to do nothing that he would refuse to do when conscious. An unscrupulous hypnotist can manipulate a subject into any situation he desires if he goes about it properly. For example, let us consider a young, religious, highly moral girl who would never, under any circumstances, willingly disrobe in front of an audience. If a clever hypnotist were to convince her that she was absolutely alone in the room and was preparing to bathe, he could have her totally naked in short order.

Equally wrong is the idea that a person cannot be hypnotized against his will. This feat is difficult and requires concerted effort on the hypnotist's part. He must avoid all mention of the word "hypnosis" or "sleep" or anything that might have a connotation of trance. A few years ago, I witnessed the hypnosis of a young girl in a classroom. She was of a religious persuasion that disallows hypnosis, and her only words as she was going under were, "You are not hypnotizing me, are you?" To this day, the girl is unaware that she was hypnotized and therefore will suffer no burden of guilt. An exploitation of this sort can only be described as unethical and reprehensible as would be the unwilling disrobing of a person in front of an audience. Fortunately for us all, these things occur very rarely and require an exceptionally skilled and devious hypnotist and a very suggestible subject.

The most widely used and advantageous application of hypnosis is that of self-hypnosis. When one hypnotizes oneself, it is virtually impossible to reach the trance state of somnambulism required, for example, for regression, as some part of the conscious mind will always be active. It is, however, relatively easy to put one's self in a depth of trance amenable to receiving helpful, supportive suggestions.

The entire emotional structure of the psyche is controlled and regulated by the unconscious mind. Almost all of our likes, dislikes and propensities are dictated by our emotions, or the unconscious. Through the application of self-hypnosis, one has a measure of control over the unconscious and, therefore, the emotional component of the mind. *When ones controls the emotional aspect of a situation, one controls the situation!*

It is extremely difficult, almost impossible, to teach oneself self-hypnosis without assistance, whereas after one has been successfully hypnotized by a professional, the procedure becomes simple. What it boils down to is merely that you are controlling the induction rather than another person. When one has once known a deep trance state, recognizes it as such, and becomes relatively familiar with it, it becomes easier to obtain said state by oneself. It is difficult to find something until you know what it is you seek.

Being extremely resistant to hypnosis, it took me longer than most to learn self-hypnosis, and several systems were used before any degree of success was attained. One night while in bed, after extensive counting (literally boring the conscious mind into oblivion), I was suddenly aware of a loud, pounding noise in my ears and realized, to my elation, that I had achieved hypnosis. The suggestion given to myself when I started counting was that I would become aware of the blood rushing through my ears.

Shortly after the blood pounding in my ears episode, I was with my daughter in a travel-trailer at a resort spa. She was asleep next to me in bed, and I was eagerly reading a new book on hypnosis I had just obtained. While reading I became suddenly and painfully aware of a cramp in my left leg. Normally when a cramp of this type hits, the only alternative is to walk around, thumping the foot against the floor. This is extremely difficult in a small travel-trailer. Because it was exactly what I happened to be reading about, I grasped at the alternative. Concentrating hard, I counted myself down into a trance, telling myself firmly that my left leg would become totally numb from the knee down. For added measure, I suggested that the sole of my left foot would become very hot. This was done only because, as I have stated, it was what I had been reading about at the time and I wanted to see if it would work. I thought the leg would become numb, but I had very little faith that the sole of my foot would become hot.

After a few minutes, I came out of the trance, was unaware of any cramp in my leg, and continued reading.

After an hour or so, deciding it was time to go to sleep, I got out of bed and headed for the bathroom—I had totally forgotten about the hypnosis. Trying to be quiet so as not to awaken my daughter, I stepped out of the bed and immediately crashed to the floor. My left leg was not working.

When my daughter awakened and asked what was happening, I told her I had numbed my leg by hypnosis. A few minutes later, I crawled into bed, and my daughter, now fully awake, demanded, "What is the world is wrong with your foot? It's red hot!" She was absolutely right; the sole of my foot was so hot one could have fried an egg on it!

Prerequisites for self-hypnosis are a strong motivation, deep concentration, diligence, and an intelligent application of suggestions.

Many persons, including myself, use self-hypnosis prior to and while visiting the dentist. This could be considered strong motivation. Any situation that involves apprehension and emotion: dental visits, surgery or painful medical treatment, court appearances, speaking before a group, etc. These situations are eased considerably by starting self-hypnosis so much as two to three days prior to the anticipated traumatic experience. It will not be totally effective if one waits until one is climbing the courthouse steps to start applying it. It should be done early, and perhaps several times prior to the situation.

While conducting my studies on twins, one of the first girls hypnotized told me she had to appear before the state legislature and give a speech. She was a nervous wreck over the prospect. The night before she was to board the plane for Sacramento, she came to see me, and, after being placed in a trance, she was given several suggestions. She was told that while on the plane, she would not even think about the upcoming talk. She would enjoy the meal served and converse with her seat mate. Further suggestions were that, after preparing the speech thoroughly (which she had already done), she would put it out of her mind until standing at the podium. Then she would single out two or three people in the front row, address her speech to them, as if she were discussing it with them in her own living room. Final suggestions were that she would remain calm, poised, and in complete control of herself throughout the entire ordeal.

A few days later, I was amused but not surprised when she called me, elated, and raved about how well the whole thing had gone. Babbling excitedly, she said, "While I was talking, I looked at two people sitting in the front row and directed my talk to them, ignoring the several hundred that were there!"

Self-hypnosis is not always an easy process, and this is why diligence is required. Learning to expel extraneous thought from the mind and to concentrate on only ONE THING is a difficult undertaking. It is especially difficult in our modern society in which we are besieged and beleaguered by telephones, television, billboards, magazines and hundreds of other distractions vying for our attention. This is one of the reasons that persons practicing meditation chant a mantra—it is an aid to concentration. Some persons picture the mind as a large blackboard, and whenever an outside thought creeps in, a large eraser comes and immediately wipes it off the board.

It has been my experience that the fastest path to hypnosis, either self or hetero, is counting. Picturing a large, never-ending staircase, one starts counting as the steps are descended. When this technique is applied consistently over a period of time (or perhaps several periods of time), eventually even the most difficult subject will enter a trance. It is similar somewhat to Esdaille's hand passes in that it is constant, repetitive and can be very time consuming. Hand passes will be discussed later.

Now we view the most important area of the hypnosis process: intelligent applications of suggestions. After all, what earthly reason is there for a person to enter a trance state if he gains nothing from the experience?

Suggestions given during self-hypnosis should be short, clear and directly to the point. It is better, particularly when first practicing self-hypnosis, to dwell upon only one suggestion, rather than confusing the unconscious with many orders and risking rejection of them all. After a particular suggestion has been decided upon, it will help to write it out on paper. Then go over it and reduce it to as short a sentence as possible. As one slowly enters the trance, a part of the conscious mind will repeat the suggestion over and over. When one has become adept at this process, the suggestions may be further reduced to one or two "key" words that, when repeated, will trigger the entire suggestion in the mind.

This brings to mind a true story about a hypnotist who frequently practiced his art on his wife. Eventually she became very conditioned to entering the trance state, and they agreed that when she heard the words "polar ice cap," she would immediately enter a state of hypnosis. They deliberately chose these words because she was unlikely to ever hear them inadvertently. One evening after a large dinner party, the wife was clearing the table of dishes and was carrying a large tray. On the radio, the newscaster stated that the U.S. Government had decided against affiliating with the Concorde airplane because of reported dangers to the "polar ice cap."

Upon hearing those three words, the poor woman immediately entered a trance, and the tray full of dishes crashed to the floor. This sort of key-word danger exists only in the hetero-hypnosis area.

It is important that everyone involved in the field of hypnosis be aware of the following statement: A suggestion, like a seed, once implanted has a propensity to become self-actuating. For this reason it is necessary that suggestions made to the unconscious mind be carefully chosen and carefully worded.

In finalizing this section on self-hypnosis, let me state that learning self-hypnosis will assist you in obtaining a good deal of mental and emotional growth. It will introduce you to areas of yourself previously undiscovered. If you use it and let it, it will add an entirely new, delightful dimension to your life.

CHAPTER SIX

CONTROLLING THE EMOTIONS WITH HYPNOSIS

THIS IS NOT A BOOK about the usual applications of hypnosis. The market is crowded with books of that type describing hypnosis for weight, smoking, etc. There are many and varied aspects of hypnosis about which little or nothing has been written and of which many practicing hypnotists fail to recognize.

When working in the field, it is important to bear one thought in mind at all times: you are limited in the use of hypnosis only so far as you are limited in your own imagination!

A few years ago I was working with a group of fairly young people who desired to quit smoking. They all worked together in an office, and when they heard about one of the group that had successfully given up cigarettes after being hypnotized by me, they all decided to try it.

One of the girls, a beautiful brunette of about twenty-four, explained that she did not smoke, that she wanted to discuss something else with me. After the group left, she explained that she was desperately in love with a man who, though he saw her on a regular basis, was not as dedicated to the affair as she was. Sobbing, she told of how she waited night after night for his call, adding that she knew he was seeing other women. This knowledge tore her up emotionally. Her overriding ambition was to marry this man, but, of course, he was having none of that.

This was a situation I had never faced before, nor had I read anything in the literature concerning problems such as this.

After explaining carefully to the girl that there were absolutely no guarantees, I calmed her down and placed her in a trance. Then she was given several suggestions to reinforce her self-image. It was pointed out to her how truly beautiful she was, how clever and intelligent she must be to have obtained and held on to a responsible job, and what a sensitive, feeling, sincere person she was. Then she was told to see the young man in question. When she nodded yes, that she was seeing him, she was further instructed to see him in very unflattering clothes—very outsized boxer shorts, ridiculous, oversized shoes, and his hair was combed in a very unflattering way. Elaborating on this idea, she was instructed to view the man in a compromising, undignified situation, such as sitting on a toilet, his large boxer shorts around his ankles. By the smile on her face it was clear this was happening. A further suggestion was given that from this point on, *he would be to her as any other man, and his emotional hold on her was broken.* When she awakened from the trance, she was clam, relaxed, and smiling.

One of the frustrating features of this work is the lack of feedback. Sometimes one sees immediate and gratifying results, such as with smoking or phantom limb pain, but many times there is no way of knowing just how successful the hypnotherapy may have been.

Nothing was heard from or about the lovely brunette for several months—no one seemed to know what the status was with her boyfriend. Then, suddenly one day I received a call from her asking me to see a friend of hers. The girl was having serious trouble because of a thwarted love affair, had a six-year-old dependent daughter, and had recently attempted suicide over the situation. The girl in trouble lived a long ways away, and because I was leaving for Europe the following morning, I tried to side-step the assignment. There were several competent hypnotists in the area where the girl lived, and it was suggested that she contact one of these. The brunette explained that because the hypnotherapy had been so overwhelmingly successful with herself (this was the first I had heard of it) that the suicidal girl insisted upon seeing me.

After a few minutes, the girl herself called and explained she had taken the day off from work and was driving over to see me. Of course I relented and agreed to work with her.

She was a redhead, every bit as strikingly beautiful as the brunette. Before we started, she was asked about the results of the hypnosis that had been used with the brunette.

Laughing, she stated, "That poor guy cannot figure out what went wrong. He asked her to go to Monaco with him a few months ago, and she refused because she did not think it would be any fun." Then she added, "Before you hypnotized her, she would have swum behind the boat all the way to Monaco just to be near him. Now she is dating several men and having a ball!"

Through her tears the lovely redhead explained that she was involved with an airline pilot who treated her very badly. After being hypnotized, she was given exactly the same suggestions as was the brunette. Awakening from the trance, she yawned, stretched, flashed a dazzling smile, and said, "I think I will make a date with that cute guy who manages the liquor store on my corner—he is always asking me."

Here is another "happy-ending" story along the same vein and absolutely true. About two years ago, my close friend, Betty, bewailed to me the problems and worries that beset her concerning her daughter, Joanie. Joanie is an only child and the light of her mother's life. Then thirty-eight years old, she held the busy, fascinating job of airline flight attendant. The problem that Joanie faced and made her mother so distraught was Joanie's husband Frank. He was a self-proclaimed artist, a n'er-do-well who had contributed nothing to the family financially. He was perfectly content to let Joanie support him.

While her mother was frantic over Frank's exploitation of her daughter, Joanie herself was ambivalent over the situation. She did not want to divorce and felt emotionally bonded to Frank. Because of his indolence and increasing drinking problem, however, her conscious, rational side demanded that she free herself from the situation.

In a quandary, and at her mother's urging, she came for hypnotherapy. The suggestions were more direct than used before. She would view her situation objectively; she would, with no emotion, set about rectifying it.

This effort took longer than it had with the two younger girls. This is probably explained by the fact that Joanie and Frank had been married several years, had a dog they both loved dearly, interweaving their lives very closely.

It took three sessions of hypnosis before Joanie calmly announced to her mother that she was leaving Frank. After two more sessions spread over a period of several months, she finally brought herself to go through with the divorce.

About five months ago she came to me and said, "I have finally met the man that should be for me. He is a few years younger, which does not bother me. His love for me is beyond measure; he has an excellent career and earns good money." She went on to describe his stability, sincerity, and other outstanding attributes. According to Joanie the only thing holding her back was the fact that she did not feel the old overwhelming impact of love that she had experienced with Frank.

It was very simple, and we did exactly what was indicated. Joanie was hypnotized and told that she would find herself, over the next few months, falling desperately in love with Jim. She would find herself hating to leave him whenever she left on a flight and that she would appreciate, more and more, all his fine qualities. Then, because she so sincerely wanted to be in love with him, it was added that she would start becoming concerned that, because he was a very eligible bachelor, some other woman might make a move on him while she was gone on one of her extended flights.

The results were astounding! A couple of weeks after the last session she announced to her mother, "I just cannot stand it when I have to leave Jim—I miss him so when I am away!" Joanie and Jim were recently married, and to all appearances are heading for a marvelous life together.

It is common knowledge that many athletes, both individually and as a team, use hypnotists. A couple of years ago, a young man who was studying scuba diving came to see me. He was, according to him, having all sorts of problems getting through the course. He explained that a lot was contingent upon him receiving his diving certificate. There was a group who was going out on the ocean searching for a specific buried treasure. They had secured maps, a ship, and the necessary financing. All that was holding up the party at that point was the young man completing his course. While he was talking, I concluded that, because he was under so much pressure to perform, he had developed a large mental block against succeeding. He knew the work, knew what was expected, but just could not manage to bring it off. Furthermore, he lacked confidence that he would ever be able to do what was required.

This, again, was something I had never tackled. As we talked, he explained to me step by step what it was he had to do, while I made notes. After assuring him that three or four sessions of hypnosis would undoubtedly restore his confidence, I placed him in a trance.

Slowly, step by step I led him through the entire procedure. He was told that he was doing everything perfectly. He could feel the coolness and buoyancy of the water, each muscle was responding on cue, that he was aware of total success and was amazed at how easy it was. From the expression on his face it was obvious that, mentally, he was experiencing a perfect dive, just as it was being described. He awoke feeling relaxed and refreshed.

That same evening about 6:00, I received a call from the young man. To say that he verged on hysteria would be an understatement. He had left the hypnosis session, gone back to the school to practice, felt so confident that he got an instructor to monitor him, and proceeded to pass the entire exam with flying colors. As he told me all this good news, he was literally screaming with excitement. This is feedback of the finest sort!

While I was studying at the university, one of the instructors told about an incident that had transpired in a previous class. It seems that there was a husband and wife team in the class. About halfway through the series, the husband asked the professor, "Do you notice anything different about Gladys?" After studying Gladys carefully for several minutes, the professor claimed that, other than looking extremely well and younger than he had thought her to be, he was stumped.

It seems that Gladys had been practicing self-hypnosis faithfully and while in a trance had mentally pictured a small, pink velvet eraser going slowly over her face and neck, lifting the tissue and erasing the wrinkles. She had followed this procedure regularly for several weeks and the results, according to the teacher, were utterly amazing. After hearing this, I filed it in my mind under the "highly questionable" category. Shortly thereafter I was discussing the classes with a friend and happened to mention the story of the improbable face lift. Her reaction was one of extreme excitement and she begged, "Oh, please try it on me!" As I was practicing hypnosis on anyone who would allow it in those days, we went ahead with it. She was a good subject, and I had her in a trance very shortly.

Dorothy (my subject) nodded yes, that she could feel the little pink eraser traveling slowly up and down, over her face and neck. She agreed that she was aware of a tightening feeling as the eraser traveled over the surface of her skin. Toward the end of the session I instructed her that in the future when she was reposed and relaxed she would mentally say the words "face lift" and the words would continue, in the days to come, to trigger all the suggestions regarding the pink eraser. She was told that as she drifted off to sleep at night and as she slowly awoke in the morning, the suggestions would be reinforced as she consciously became aware of the words "face lift."

After the meeting with Dorothy I became busy moving out into the country and completely forgot what we had done. It had left my head immediately because I could think of absolutely no reason why anything seemingly this ridiculous should work.

It was several months before I saw Dorothy again. She arrived at my home one afternoon to spend the weekend. Upon arrival she complained of a ferocious headache, caused by freeway traffic, so I suggested that she lay down for a few minutes and let me help her to relax. After a few suggestions about muscles and arteries in her head relaxing, she was completely pain free. During the course of the relaxation procedure I subconsciously noticed how glowing and youthful her skin looked. Giving it no more thought, I brought her out of the light trance and we immediately left to keep an appointment. Much later that evening as we were having dinner in a restaurant, a friend observed, "Dorothy, I have never seen you looking so good. You look twenty years younger than when I first met you."

Suddenly a light went on in my head and I looked at her in amazement and said, "The little pink eraser!"

Dorothy giggled and admitted that she had, indeed, been practicing the pink eraser routine with amazing results. If I had not personally observed this phenomenon with my own eyes, I never would have believed it.

As stated earlier, the unconscious mind shows elements of powerful autonomy. Occasionally a hypnotist will use a pendulum on a chain to communicate with the unconscious. The pendant is dangled between the thumb and first finger and allowed to swing freely. It is soon learned that the pendant will swing correspondingly with an image in the mind. If one thinks about or mentally pictures a circle, for instance, soon the pendulum will swing in a circle. If one pictures a larger circle, the pendulum will swing more widely, with absolutely no movement or control of the supporting hand or fingers. A subject readily learns to make the pendant swing in a circle, back and forth from the body and crosswise with the body. A set of signals is established, back and forth to mean negative and crosswise to signal yes, or affirmative.

Interesting conversations can be conducted with a person holding a pendulum both in the hypnotic trance or fully conscious. When working with a person in the conscious state, it is advisable to prop a piece of cardboard or a magazine in such a way so that the person involved cannot see the pendulum.

One afternoon I was talking to a friend of my daughter. She had just learned how to use the pendulum but could not see the one she was holding. Francis had just enrolled herself in nurses training and was telling me all about it. When I asked if she really thought she was going to enjoy nursing, she babbled excitedly, "Oh, yes, it's something I have wanted to do all my life!"

There is an interesting highlight to this story. All the time Francis was raving animatedly about her future nursing career, the pendulum was swinging steadily and firmly in the "no" response. Finally I removed the cardboard cover and showed her what was happening. The look on her face was a real study! Complete and total amazement and surprise. Francis continued with her course, became a registered nurse and then discovered she could not abide nursing. Last word from her was that she had applied and been accepted to medical school and would become a doctor.

There are fascinating answers to a lot of life's problems buried in the unconscious mind if we choose to take the time to find them. Some are fairly obvious and some are not so obvious.

One evening, after I had first started studying hypnosis, I was enjoying cocktails with a group of friends, and the subject of the book *Paradise Lost* was raised. We were all trying to remember who the author was. Right there in the bar I quickly hypnotized myself and suggested that the author's name would come to me. Probably somewhere in the neighborhood of fifty years had passed since I had studied English literature and *Paradise Lost.* It was much later, during the dessert course of dinner, that I suddenly hollered to the surprised group, "John Milton!" A startled friend on my right asked, "Who's he?" and I quickly explained that he was the author of *Paradise Lost.*

CHAPTER SEVEN

CONFIDENCE

IT WAS SEVERAL YEARS before I became interested in hypnosis that the awesome power of the unconscious mind was portrayed to me in a somewhat obtuse fashion. It was back a few years ago when terrariums were in vogue. As half owner in a giftware manufacturing company, I designed a new line of merchandise called driftwood candles. These were sand candles built around "driftwood" which was really old, dead grapevines pulled off the fields by our workers. After the grapes were harvested, the growers were delighted to have us come in and clear the old vines off the fences. The driftwood candles were a beautiful, simple, extremely high-profit item which were rapidly catching on in the market place.

After we had been in production for a few months, suddenly we were faced with what appeared to be an insurmountable problem. Several persons had purchased the candles as gift items, had them ornately wrapped, and had presented them for weddings, birthdays, etc.

The problem surfaced when the gift recipient opened the box bearing the candle to find it crawling with termites, spiders and other forms of insect life. During the manufacture of the candles they were dipped at least once in hot paraffin, but this was not, obviously, enough to kill insects or eggs that were imbedded in the wood.

We were faced with a host of unhappy merchandisers, and our candles were rapidly being banned from better stores on the West Coast.

My partner and I racked our brains as to how best to handle the crisis. He finally decided to get a vat of formaldehyde and soak the wood in it for a few days prior to making candles. I begged him to wait a while before taking this radical step as it would present many production problems, not the least of which was the fire hazard and the serious delay in production.

At that particular time, my son was enrolled in a pre-medical course at the University of California at Irvine, and because it was during the summer break, he was residing with me.

A few weeks earlier he had been describing to me the intricacies of the microwave oven while I was preparing dinner for him one evening. As I had plans for the evening, I was paying absolutely no attention to what he was saying.

When the problems at the giftware company reached crisis proportions, I realized that I had to come up with an answer if I was to dissuade my partner from going the formaldehyde route. That night I went to sleep with this problem on my mind, and the next morning when I awoke, the answer was there, crystal clear.

Calling my partner, I advised him to stop on the way to the factory and pick up a microwave oven. Then we directed the wood cutters to cut the grapevines a certain length. When about fifteen or twenty sticks were cut, they were placed into the oven, and it was run for about forty-five seconds to a minute. We could watch through the glass window in the front. The bugs would immediately leave the wood; then they would blow up. The eggs harbored in the wood were quickly destroyed, and the wood was cool and bug-free when removed from the oven. This proved to be a clean, quick, and highly efficient answer to a serious problem. An answer that, when given a chance, sifted up from the depths of my unconscious mind.

The unconscious mind is literal to the extreme. This is why the proper phrasing of suggestions to a hypnotized person is so important. Innuendo simply does not work. One may say to a person in trance, "Can you tell us what you are seeing?" and the reply will be a simple "Yes." He *can* tell you, but unless so instructed, he will not. The proper phraseology is, "As you view these things, you *will* describe to us what you are seeing."

Persons in the trance state are inordinately susceptible to suggestions of all sorts. This includes persons under anesthesia as well as those under hypnosis.

A registered nurse who was in one of my hypnosis classes told about an incident that occurred at the hospital where she worked. She was on duty in the operating room when the following happened. Surgery was in progress; the patient was being operated upon for a bleeding stomach ulcer. A young nurses' aid entered the room carrying several glass jars of whole blood. The jars of blood slipped from her hand and crashed to the floor. When this happened, she screamed, "Oh, my God, there's blood everywhere!" The man undergoing surgery immediately started to hemorrhage and before the doctor could stem the flow, the patient bled to death.

When a person is in a state of hypnosis, his senses are keen and hyperacute. This fact was portrayed to me very clearly a few years ago. A young friend of my daughter's was having problems at work. At the time she was twenty-two years old and had been promoted to forelady over a group of about fifteen women who were all twice her age or more. While she was hypnotized, I gave her strong suggestions about her own worth, about retaining her sense of humor, and most of all about how she would be strong and forceful when the occasion demanded it. Then I ended the suggestions by telling her that she would have the fortitude to fire any of the women who failed to recognize her authority or show her proper respect.

Before the session began, the telephone had been removed from the hook in the kitchen and two doors were closed between the kitchen and bedroom to insure privacy. About one-half way through the session, the telephone suddenly jangled loudly in the kitchen. My subject remained unperturbed, but it scared the day-lights out of me and I jumped perceptibly.

When I brought my subject out of the trance, she laughed and remarked, "When the phone rang, it scared the wits out of you, didn't it?" She went on to explain that while hypnotized she had heard the car drive into the driveway, heard the key go into the lock, heard my daughter Evie come into the house and replace the phone on its hook. This was fascinating to me because, although my hearing is excellent, I heard none of these things as they happened.

The same young woman, whom I shall call Sharon (she gave me permission to use her pictures, but she prefers I not use her real name), came to see me at a later time.

Her work was going fine, she said; the suggestions regarding confidence and her ability to lead had taken hold, and she had a firm grip on the situation at work.

However, she was feeling depressed, had no love life to speak of, and she was lonely. Sharon was tall, lithe, and possessed a gorgeous figure which she kept carefully hidden under jeans and baggy T-shirts. Her dull, lifeless dishwater blond hair hung limply about her face, which, despite excellent bone structure, was sallow and colorless. Her eyes were dull, probably from boredom.

Inspired, I asked, "Sharon, how about putting yourself in my hands for a couple of weeks?" Surprised, she inquired what I intended to do. "Just wait and see, " I answered.

Sharon came by twice a week after work for a couple of weeks. First I would hypnotize her and feed her self-confidence sugges-tions. Then we lightened her hair three or four shades and colored it. On her next visit, we went shopping, and she bought a matching hair piece and a lot of various cosmetics. Then a sexy new cocktail dress to wear to the upcoming factory party, along with some high-heeled sandals and a clever evening bag.

A few days later I gave her lessons on applying the makeup, foundation, blusher, and things to highlight the eyes. Later I showed her various ways to fix her hair, some integrating the

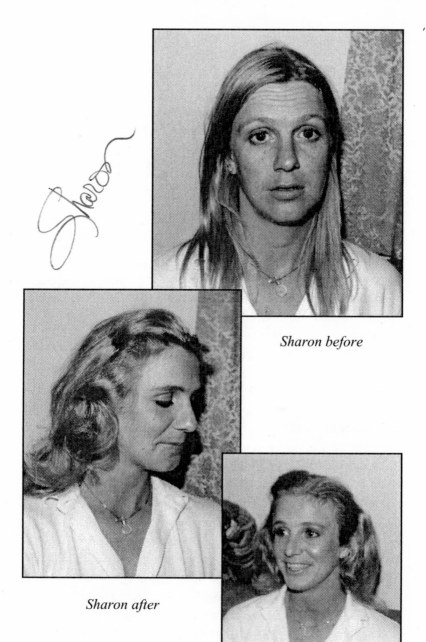

Sharon before

Sharon after

hairpiece. The accompanying pictures portray the transformation. Our duckling turned into a swan!

On the night of the big party I met Sharon at her apartment. We fixed her hair in a glamorous upsweep, carefully applied the makeup, put on the dazzling cocktail dress, shoes and—WOW! There was droopy, lifeless little Sharon, looking for all the world like a movie star!

I had worked on her posture and carriage and her attitude with hypnosis. Shoulders back, head held high, she looked, acted, and walked like a queen.

When Sharon entered the banquet hall that night, everything ground to a halt. All eyes were upon her. She walked casually and gracefully to the bar and ordered a drink. Immediately she was besieged from all sides. The girls demanded to know how she had pulled off this miracle, and the boys wanted to know where she had been hiding all this time?

The frosting on the cake was when the company president walked over and invited her to sit at his table.

Within a matter of weeks Sharon had been promoted off the production line into the office. Promotions continued, and a few years ago, when the company opened a plant in South America, she was one of the lucky ones chosen to oversee the plant's development and opening.

After several years of hard work, going to school nights, she obtained a college degree. Today she is married, has an outstanding top-level job, and is one happy woman!

An animal that feels threatened or perceives danger will immediately enter a catatonic state similar to hypnosis. Its actions will freeze and every sense appears to be hyperalert.

A consensus among neurologists is that the center controlling hypnosis is located in an atavistic area of the brain, and it is reasonable to assume that at one time man used something similar to hypnosis as do animals today, to perceive danger. Through the process of evolution, this trait obviously became repressed, more so in some than others. Perhaps this explains why some people are more readily hypnotized than others.

The human mind, like the human body, has an inherent tendency to heal itself when ill. Practicing psychologists and psychiatrists soon become aware that the mind also has a strong self-protective instinct and will shut down when a threat becomes too great. Persons in a catatonic trance have simply turned themselves off to unbearable outside stimuli, either physical or mental. Women who have been subjected to gang rape invariably tell the same story, i.e., "After a while it was as if it was happening to someone else. I felt like I was up near the ceiling and that stranger on the floor was undergoing the abuse, not myself." When it is functioning properly, this mental protective aspect helps persons endure untold hardships and horror.

More common is the day-by-day, slowly growing, insidious trauma that brings people to the breaking point. It is when we feel ourselves trapped in frustrating, unrewarding situations to which no end is in sight that we become suicidal or break down. Barbara, a friend of mine, was a person in such a situation. She begged me to help her through hypnosis and again, having no idea whether or not it would work, I agreed to try.

Barbara is among the legions of persons in our society trying to adjust to a colostomy. At least this is what she blamed for her state of mind when we started working together. However, many other facts revealed themselves during the course of several interviews. Upon selling their fairly large home, Barbara and her husband had moved to a rural community and into a narrow mobile home. None of this was Barbara's idea; it had been pushed on her by her husband. Like most couples who have been married many years, there was no excitement left in their marriage, if indeed there ever had been any. Barbara felt trapped in a hopeless situation. She abhorred the idea of the colostomy and could not reconcile to it. She hated the community in which she found herself because it lacked the sophistication of the large city. She hated the small, crowded unaesthetic mobile home she found herself living in, but most of all, whether she acknowledged it or not, she resented her husband with a vehement passion!

During the initial interview, she made no effort to conceal her suicidal tendencies, explaining that death, to her, was preferable to the way she was currently living.

After several sessions of hypnosis, Barbara learned to view her situation differently. She, herself, is a warm, friendly, thoroughly charming person who makes friends easily. She was urged to get out of the house as much as possible.

Volunteer work at the local hospital has made a new person out of her. Thanks to hypnosis, she now views her dull husband as an old and faithful friend. Energy formally expended in condemning Charles and her situation is now spent in the many activities she sought and found. Though her life is far from ideal, she has learned to adjust and cope with it the best possible way.

The unconscious mind keeps a record of everything we have ever seen, heard, felt, or experienced. It is as though there were a never-ending video tape running somewhere in our brain. A person, when hypnotized, can be regressed to any point in his life. This may be handled in one of two ways: the subject can actually regress mentally into a given point in his past. He will sometimes assume the characteristics of that age and will actually, in his mind, relive the era. There have been cases in my own experience when I have regressed people into infancy and found that they respond to the Babinski test with an infantile reaction. When the sole of an adult's foot is stroked a certain way, he will respond by arching his foot downward. An infant will jerk his foot so the toe points upward towards his knee. This is known as the Babinski reflex. The other way to regress a person is to have him only "view" the period objectively. This latter system is more efficient when gleaning facts about a particularly traumatic experience. One is able to learn exactly what happened without the accompanying emotion. It should be noted here that this is not always the simple procedure that it may appear to be. Regression demands a somnambulistic state of trance, and many persons require a lengthy induction, or several inductions, before achieving the required depth of trance.

This system of recall has proven especially beneficial in police investigations. One of the more notorious of these transpired several years ago in Chowchilla, California, when a school bus full of children was hijacked. The bus driver and children finally managed to escape. Later the driver and a witness were hypnotized by Dr. William Kroger. Under hypnosis they were able to provide police with a description of the vans driven by the abductors along with descriptions of the kidnappers and partial license plate numbers. Armed with this information, the police were able to arrest and later convict the culprits.

Several years ago, a friend of my daughter's was raped. She developed complete amnesia after the act, could give police no clue as to the description of the man. Shortly thereafter, she asked if I would hypnotize her. This I did and directed her to view the entire process, detached and unemotionally.

She proceeded to describe exactly how the man had broken into her apartment, physically overcame her while threatening her with a knife. Then she described him minutely—his race, size, approximate weight, clothing, jewelry, ending with a description of an extra-large belt buckle he wore. She delivered the tape to the police, and I understand that shortly thereafter the man was arrested.

A man of about forty came to me a while back and asked my help. He stated that he wished to discover why there had always existed an emotional barrier between himself and his father. He said, "I have always felt that my father rejected me. He never gave me the love he showed my brother. Many times he treated me as a stranger."

When he was adequately hypnotized, the man was instructed to regress in time to a period in his youth when he had done something pleasant with his father. It was suggested that perhaps they were fishing together or viewing a sports event.

His terse statement surprised me. Through clenched teeth, he explained, "He's not my father!" Taken aback, I inquired why he believed that. "Because he said so," was the answer. He was instructed to go to the time when he first became aware the man claimed not to be his father.

He described a small boy of three dressed in pajamas with feet in them, huddled at the top of a staircase. There was a heated verbal battle transpiring below between the parents. Then he heard the man accuse the woman of infidelity, finally hollering that the boy was not his son. His mother was saying nothing, just sitting on the sofa sobbing. When told to advance a half hour in time, he said that the man had stormed out of the house, slamming the door. The woman remained on the sofa, crying.

Instructing him that he would remember everything he had seen and heard, I brought him back to the conscious state. Immediately it was explained to him that even though he had heard his father make the statement that the boy was not his issue, this did not mean that it was necessarily true. He agreed with this and added, "It does not matter. It isn't important if I am his son or not. What is important is that now I know the basis for his attitude towards me." This was something that had bothered him all of his life, and he was very relieved to finally have an answer.

This brings to mind a similar, more recent incident. One morning I received a call from a Swedish woman. She was in this country visiting her daughter who was an exchange student. While talking to a Swedish friend of mine, she had heard about an extensive study into regression I had done regarding a queen born in Sweden in 1626. The study fascinated her, and she insisted on meeting with me. After we had finished discussing the regression research, she asked me to hypnotize her. Her grandparents were both dead, and she wished to see them again, and she added something about seeing her father. When she was in trance, I regressed her back to her childhood so she could relive time spent with her beloved grandparents. Then, to her dismay, I brought her out of the trance. She beseeched me to rehypnotize her, stating, "It's my father; it's something about my father." I assumed he was dead from her vague statements.

Again back into her childhood, she was viewing her parents. While she was describing them, I was sitting with my eyes closed, mentally viewing the people she was describing. When she finished with her mother, she started delineating her father. She started by saying he was very tall. Because I was receiving a clear mental picture of the man, I interjected, "He has blond hair, dark blond." She agreed and went on to state that it was straight and combed back to the side. Then she continued, saying that his eyes were an unusual blue color. I added, "like turquoise," and she readily agreed. We both concurred that he was a handsome, clean-cut, blond, blue-eyed man. Then, suddenly a very peculiar expression swept over her face, and she inquired, "Why am I lying here, saying my father is a blue-eyed blond man, when I know he has dark hair and eyes?" Stumped for an answer, I brought her out of the trance. Her state of bewilderment was genuine, and she was very concerned about what we had both seen.

Let me interject a thought here. After working in hypnosis through the years, it has been my discovery that I am experiencing more and more psychic phenomena. Many times I am able to mentally picture what a person is seeing in their mind—what they are seeing or feeling before they express it. There seems to develop a psychic interaction between subject and hypnotist. This happens only occasionally.

There was no way to explain to the woman why she had envisioned the blond man as her father. Likewise, there was no rational explanation as to why she had been so obsessed with seeing her father under hypnosis, particularly when the man she called father was still living. Possibly she had an unconscious speculation that that man was not, in fact, her real father.

The only thing I could think of was to suggest to her, half laughingly, that perhaps she should have a heart-to-heart talk with her mother upon returning home. One thing struck me later (and this I did not call to her attention) was the striking similarity of her teenage daughter to the man we had both seen in our minds, especially the girl's eyes, which were the same turquoise blue as the man we had envisioned.

CHAPTER EIGHT

A CLOSE LOOK AT HOMOSEXUALITY

PREVIOUS REFERENCES HAVE BEEN MADE to regression work with a "Swedish Queen" and research on identical twins and triplets. Allow me to elaborate on these studies in order to lay groundwork for disclosures to come.

Several years ago, I conducted some past-life regressions merely in an exploratory vein. My first subject was Marcia Simpson, then thirty-two, of Garden Grove, California. Marcia regressed into the life of a queen that was born in Sweden in 1626. As stated earlier she gave the name "Priscilla." Later it was discovered that the queen's name had been Christina. Through the course of several years of regressions, Marcia portrayed for me the entire life of this colorful woman.

Sometimes (depending upon who was addressing her) she understood Swedish and French upon hearing it spoken to her. She seemed to have related better to men, although it was a woman who spoke to her in French—which she appeared to understand fairly easily. Marcia, in trance, identified pictures of the queen's parents and all the members of her court, including some little known ones. Likewise she recognized and named pictures of Louis XIV and other outstanding personalities of the time. She was able to describe with absolute accuracy hundreds of events that occurred during the life of Christina. We must realize that very little has been translated about this queen into English. Most of the personal events that she described have never been translated into English, and many of them are generally unknown today, even to the average Swede. One instance is that Marcia referred frequently to the queen's older brother. Christina did, in fact, have an illegitimate half-brother ten years her senior of which a lot of historians are unaware. It is my firm belief that these past-life memories (everyone has them), form the basis of our personality. Through them is developed our basic intelligence level, our propensities, talents, attitudes, and disposition. This explains why two children close in age, raised in an entirely identical environment, can be exact opposites. Any woman who has raised two or more children will acknowledge this fact.

Therefore, I further contend, a study of a person's past-life memories can be extremely revealing. In these memories may lie the key to today's phobias, compulsions, obsessions, talents, and even sexual orientation.

When my daughter Evie was almost eight years old, she was home one day when the house burned down. Even though the neighbor who was watching her got her out safely, the fire seemed to have been an inordinately traumatic experience for her. A while back we decided to hypnotize her in an effort to discover why this was so.

In the trance, she was advised to revert back to a lifetime when fire had been an important factor. As she was counted down into the trance, I watched as her face contorted, being totally unprepared for what followed. Suddenly she gasped and in utter anguish, she choked out the words, "They are all dead; all the children are dead!" Tears were streaming down her face. After she was calmed down and ordered to just view the event, she was able to tell the following story: The setting was a Welsh mining town (Evie has a strong Welsh heritage), and she saw herself as a thirty-two-year-old woman who looked "olderly." (This meant that the woman looked older than her years.) The woman, who was a widow, was cooking dinner for her three children, two, five, and seven. She had stepped out to the market to get something, and she returned to find her house in flames, all the children dead from the smoke. She explained how the houses are built to follow the contours of the hills, built into the ground for insulation. The room containing the children was above the kitchen and inaccessible. Something had been cooking in the oven (later, when conscious, she elaborated that it was an open-hearth type of oven), and a coal had jumped into the room igniting the house.

Several other houses had also burned, resulting in deaths other than her three children. She felt that the father had most likely died in a mine accident. When asked how long the woman had lived, she answered in a strong, tremulous voice, fraught with emotion, "She died that day!" Elaborating, she explained that the woman had been both devastated and destroyed in spirit that day and had died by her own hand a short while after the fire.

This story explains why a certain song always brings Evie to tears. It is a song by a group called "The Byrds." The name of the song is "The Bells of Rhyme." It is a song about a Welsh mining tragedy and, unbeknownst to her, it was reigniting the whole tragic incident.

When Evie heard the tape of this story while conscious, she said that there had been another lifetime when fire had been important. A few days later she was rehypnotized and, shaking a clenched fist, a look of total animation on her face, she hollered, "Burn, burn!"

This life was that of a young man (who looked, she added, like her brother, Conly, today) who was active during the French Revolution. He was tall, slender with dark blond hair—in his mid-twenties. His clothing was that of the lesser nobility, black knee pants, white socks up to his knees, white ruffled shirt. She kept repeating, "We're even burning our own homes!" The look on her face was one of elated animation and excitement as she continued to describe the utter chaos of the revolution. The young French man had had a much happier life than the pathetic Welsh widow. After the revolution, his land had been restored to him, and he eventually married, had children, and led a relatively peaceful life.

Evie spoke of another lifetime in France when she had been a concert pianist. She was an intellectual and a political activist. Eventually soldiers caught her and mutilated her hands, eventually chopping them off. That person had made his living with his hands. At the time when this story came out, Evie was a drummer in a band, and her primary career was that of master machinist. She had always been very paranoid about her hands, clenching them a lot and holding them close to her. She was inordinately concerned about injury to them. Now she understands the underlying concern.

The more study I have devoted to these past-life memories that we all have hidden in the recesses of our minds, the more convinced I become of their power to influence our present-day lives. It is my opinion that beyond a doubt, these archetypes of the past affect our sexual orientation.

Perhaps a young man who today finds himself geared toward homosexuality might regress back into the life of a well-adjusted female. Most likely the woman would be one who thoroughly enjoyed being a woman, was comfortable in her femininity and secure in her sexuality. This might explain the man's inability to gear himself exclusively to an all-masculine role in this life. At first glance this rationale appears to be sound and plausible. The only trouble is that it does not develop that way.

Over a period of several months, I regressed about thirty-five homosexual men and women. To my surprise, when instructed to regress into past lives that influence their present sexual orientation, they all regressed right back into homosexual lifetimes—the men into masculine lives and the women into lesbian lives. Many of them did, however, regress back into gay lives of the opposite sex.

This is not to infer that gay persons regress back into exclusively gay lifetimes. They are all capable of reverting back into many heterosexual eras. It is only when directed towards lives that have influenced their present-day preference that they will mirror their current proclivities.

Some of these past-life memories reflected by the gay people were extremely enlightening and clarifying. They all told of extreme persecution and of the terror of being found out for what they were. A very large number, both men and women, described lives of so-called celibacy in the Catholic Church. According to them, the homosexual life was simpler as a priest or nun. They faced none of the ubiquitous pressure to marry, and the homosexual lifestyle was easier to protect under the cloak of Catholicism.

It was my experience that the homosexual group is anxious to cooperate with anyone researching the "whys" of homosexuality. When asked to participate in the study, their primary concern was whether or not I was going to attempt to alter or "cure" their homosexuality. None were interested in going that route. Most of them had been to psychiatrists to placate their parents, and some with disastrous results.

One fact became very clear to me as I talked to these young people. No one chooses to be gay. They all felt that they had been born gay and had no choice in the matter. All of them had cousins or uncles or other close relatives that they either knew or suspected to be gay. Most had tried heterosexual relationships which they found totally unrewarding. As one young man stated, "It was as though I were committing an unnatural act."

Homosexuality seems to be something in the intrinsic makeup, an innate part of the personality, a part that defies change, not that most desire change. It is as much a part of them as their hair color or body build. A person can change his hair color, but it is a surface change; underneath the hair remains the original color.

The homosexual is not born sick; he is born different from the norm. It is society with its condemnation that makes him sick. My opinion is that it is the balance of past-life memories that dictates and controls one's sexuality.

Several of my subjects said they had been sexually molested as children, but they did not feel that the abuse had any bearing on them being gay.

A few of my subjects were able to view past lifetimes of happy heterosexual liaisons, but for the most part they reverted to strongly homosexual lives or lives of confusion, repression, or unhappy heterosexual experiences.

For the most part, the lives described were those of colorless individuals who were not distinguished other than they were gay people, generally very frustrated and unfulfilled. Some of the stories told to me were unusual, and some were pretty far-fetched. Following are some of those stories.

One young woman described the life of a woman who lived in medieval times. The woman was a psychic, maybe a witch, and commanded a lot of respect. She worked with herbs, was a healer. The witch was a homosexual, and my subject concluded, "She influences my current interest in chemistry." The subject then was instructed to describe another life wherein chemistry was a factor. It was a man, an American Indian who was a witch doctor and healer who again used herbs. Living in the American southwest, he was also a homosexual but very repressed. He recognized his feelings, but social pressures of the tribe absolutely prohibited any expression on his part. He used to watch the young men and admire their bodies, thought they were beautiful. He had to be extremely discreet even in this, as an open homosexual would never be tolerated in the village.

Another young lesbian reverted to a man, living in India, an Indian man. He had a younger lover and was not accepted by the villagers. The subject was of English heritage and said the Indian man was related to her today through a distant relative who had been stationed in India. The native had been a craftsman who fashioned pots and made rope. Her next lifetime was of a young

French girl, very pretty, who was married with children. She was very bored and only tolerated sex with her husband, much preferring women. She was popular and had many friends and one female lover. Her husband suspected her actions but tolerated it because he loved her.

The subject told of yet another life of an older, unmarried woman who lived alone in London. She worked as a practical nurse and had a very austere life. Her only satisfaction in life was helping people. She was a very plain woman who did not allow herself to think about sex, but if she had, she most certainly would have been homosexual. The woman was a great aunt of the hypnotized subject, an aunt the subject said she had never met.

One young man saw himself in the year 1940. He was a twenty-five-year-old German who was half Jewish. He was also an overt homosexual who worked for the government. When it was discovered that he was partly Jewish and a homosexual, he was put in a camp and later killed. He told of lining up with other men, ostensibly to go into the "showers," but he knew it was a gas chamber. His description of the pellets being thrown in from trap doors in the ceiling was chillingly real.

Another young man said he found himself on a boat. He was off the coast of Sweden, about 1200 A.D., dressed in skins and holding a spear. There were about twelve or fifteen men on the boat which was high in the front and back. The men were all very big, over six feet tall. He was on a trapping trip, after skins and furs. They were going to an island. His name was Sven, and he was a tanner who made a good living. He had a nice home in Sweden where he lived with another man, his lover. As a child he had had a pet goat, and when it died, his father taught him how to tan so he could always have his pet with him. That was how he learned the trade.

In another life, the same subject saw himself as an army pilot in 1942; he flew single-engine fighter planes. When asked if he was in the Air Force, he was quick to correct, "No, it's the Army Air Corps" (which is absolutely correct).

The young man was killed in a plane crash in the South Pacific. He was not a happy man, was maladjusted sexually.

Next we talked to a male homosexual. He described a life in Germany in the 1800s where he worked as a carpenter's apprentice, an artisan. He was homosexual but refused to discuss it. The repressive mores of the time inhibited any discussion of this type, he stated. Then he told about a life in France a few hundred years ago. He was a scholar, a philosopher, writing with a quill pen— fancy writing, big swirls. The man had written many books, mostly about law. He was a dull, uninteresting person who had an unhappy marriage and one child. When this subject was told to go into a strong heterosexual life in his background, he said, "I know him; it's my grandfather. He's posing for a photograph. The woman to his left is my grandmother when she was younger, and the other woman looks like my mother."

My next subject was a male homosexual. He told of a life of a nun of French descent living in New York early in the 1900s. She was asexual, had no desire to marry. His next life was a different nun who was overtly lesbian. She belonged to a large group of nuns who were all homosexual. Of course the church was unaware of this. At age thirty-five, she had been sent to a small church in Maine, and a few years later, she was still in Maine. She had established a sexual liaison with a young girl in the town. It was a very happy life, but unfortunately she was killed accidentally shortly thereafter. This young man stated that at age twenty-two in this life, he had experienced an overpowering urge to join the Catholic Church and become a priest—had actually started the wheels in motion to do it. He has no known Catholic background and has had very little exposure to the Catholic religion or church in this life.

Another male homosexual told the following story when re-gressed: "I am on a throne, lots of men around me. A woman just walked by; she is very upset because I am here with the men. She is very jealous; she is intended to be my wife." He described himself as fat with rust-colored hair and beard; his eyes are greenish with flecks of rust, and he was of medium height. He continued that he was not married at the present, that he had had a wife, but he had her killed. The year was around 1500; he was in England and was royalty. His sexual preference was definitely for men, always had been, and he fought to keep it secret. "When someone finds out, they have to be disposed of." Feeling he had to protect his image, he consorted with women to cover up. Very few people knew that he was bisexual, predominantly homosexual. His life was devoted to finding a woman he could trust to know his real preference and not betray him, one who would pose as his wife in name only, except to bear children. The man, who was obviously Henry VIII, he concluded, was not religious at all; he merely used religion to get his way. He closed with "There is one young man, Lester, sitting down there (gestures) of whom I am very fond."

A young lesbian reverted to the life of a witch in 1540 whose name was Alvia. She cast spells and was generally very unpopular. People were frightened of her. Alvia was basically a lesbian but kept to herself. The subject was reticent to discuss the life of Alvia, kept repeating, "She was rotten!" She claimed that when the witch cast a spell on someone, they usually died. The end of her life was spent in prison, and eventually she was burned at the stake. When in the conscious state, she said that it upset her to see the life of Alvia, that the woman had been very evil. There were things in the life of the witch she did not wish to think about or talk about, that maybe she had murdered some babies.

The conclusion to this section on homosexuality is the story a male homosexual told when regressed. He saw himself in biblical times as a man about twenty-five years old, medium height, dark hair and eyes and dark complexion. He's talking to a man with long hair. "I love him very much." When asked if the man was his lover, he answered an adamant, "no." The other man was definitely not homosexual. The long-haired man was about to die. "He makes all sorts of outlandish claims, and they are about to kill him. I love him, but he is about to get us all killed." The subject was getting very upset so I took him ahead two years. He said the friend had been crucified, that he was Christ. He said that he had been Christ's friend for a long time, that his name was Judas. "I had to betray Christ to save the rest of us. Christ knows that I am an avowed homosexual, and so is Peter, but he loves us anyway. I try to be discreet about it, but Peter is more open." Judas was a very jealous person, especially when he did not get the attention he wanted. After Christ's death, he had felt so guilty he hung himself.

CHAPTER NINE

LIFE IN THE WOMB

ONE OF THE MOST PERTINENT ISSUES facing our society today is the abortion issue. Just how much of an individual is that unborn child? Is the fetus an individual at all or merely an extension of the mother's body? When does life and awareness really begin?

Some of the most interesting and intriguing areas of hypnotic research I have conducted have been listening to people relive and experience their time in the womb.

Learned persons have challenged this, asking, "How can an infant or an unborn fetus think and talk and put ideas into words?"

This is a point well taken, and the answer is that we do not think, or even dream, at the unconscious level in terms of language. We think in terms of symbols; language is an acquired skill.

The biggest obstacle encountered in these types of hypnotic regressions is the problem of semantics. Subjects in a somnambulistic state sometimes find it exceedingly difficult to communicate their feelings and impressions. As we go back further into Jung's "collective unconscious," we encounter problems in labeling. For instance, a weapon or instrument that was used in Sweden in 1600 most certainly had a valid Swedish name for which there may be no English counterpart today. Therefore the subject can only describe the item, while seeking the name in frustration.

It is my personal opinion that all infants are born in a state of total hypnosis, the conscious mind forming slowly in the early years of life.

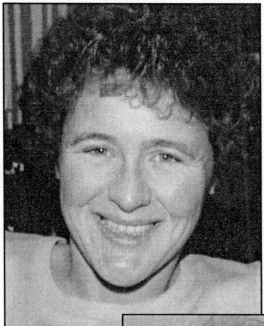

Evie Rieder, who features heavily in many of the author's hypnosis experiments

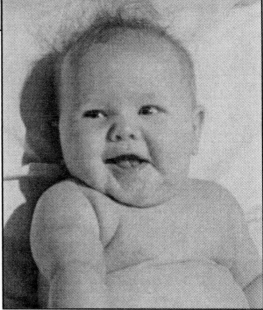

Baby Evie Rieder at two and a half months, looking none the worse for wear despite an extremely traumatic birth

At the termination of my twin and triplet study, I brought two of the triplets through their birth experience individually and at separate times and places. Their stories were identical, each describing the birth as the other had. They were particularly aware of the metallic clang of the instruments being dropped on a tray while still in utero. After the birth, they told of being in an incubator in the nursery while they watched their excited father cry and hug the doctor. Later they were all three in their mother's arms when the flash of a photographer's bulb shocked them. At this point in their story, both of the girls, tears streaming down their faces, informed me, "Dad leaned over Mom and he said—he said—I love you."

Even more interesting was my last session with one of the Morgan twins. He had asked if he could bring his wife to witness our last session, and I had readily agreed. As I brought him back towards the present time after regression, it was decided to have him relive his birth. This was not done with his brother or the third triplet simply because it had not occurred to me.

After giving him extensive suggestions that he was in the womb and the birth process had begun and he was being propelled towards the birth canal, I sensed that this was not happening. No response at all other than a rapid eye movement and the statement, "There's stuff floating by." He repeated several times that he was aware of the amniotic fluid passing by him, and the R.E.M. (rapid eye movement) continued. Try as I might, I was unable to elicit any response that denoted the birth process. From the corner of my eye, my peripheral vision told me that his wife, who was sitting near the foot of the couch, was becoming extremely amused by the proceedings. Finally, I became disgusted and told him that he was right at the moment of birth, and what was he seeing and experiencing?

Nearly jumping off the sofa, he exclaimed loudly, "There's a BRIGHT light!"

Immediately after I had brought him slowly up out of the trance, his extremely amused wife questioned of me, "Didn't you know that these boys were delivered by Caesarian section?"

This incident most certainly argues the point that many psychologists make, that is, that a hypnotized person will invariably assume the role that the hypnotist directs him to, be it true or not.

The case of my own daughter's birth was much different than any of the others as, of course, I was very subjectively involved. It was done in two separate hypnosis sessions, staged some time apart. At the first meeting, she was brought forward from the fifth month up through the birth. She told me later that she had had an awareness of the baby before the fifth month, so at another time we went from the fifth month slowly backwards all the way to her observation of the eggs in the ovary.

From these studies I learned several things about her birth of which I had been unaware. The delivery was one of the most trying that the doctor had ever attended, and he was extremely hesitant to discuss it with me when it was over. One statement I do recall him making, however, is that the baby fought him every inch of the way while he was attempting to turn her.

It has always been my misconception that the fetus became tangled in the cord during the birth process. As you read on you will learn, as I did, that this was not the case. Nor was I aware that the infant's feet and legs had protruded and had been replaced by the doctor, but I immediately recalled the state of panic that ensued in the delivery room after this happened—people rushing about, trays being wheeled in and suddenly the room seemed full of people!

When I first suggested hypnosis to my daughter, her reaction was negative. She felt that because I was her mother, it would be impossible for me to hypnotize her. After I retaliated with a statement to the effect that she should humor me and let me try, she readily agreed. Incidentally now, much later, she feels that these sessions and others we have had have helped her immeasurably to understand herself.

As I suspected, she turned out to be an excellent subject and almost immediately regressed to her seventh birthday, which she described to me as accurately as I can recall. Then I took her back to her second Christmas, to an incident that I do vividly recall but that I knew she could have no conscious memory of. While describing the toys under the tree, suddenly her face became animated, and she exclaimed, "My chair—my little blue rocking chair!"

Then she went on to relive and relate an incident that had occurred with her brother, Conly, who was then five. He wanted the chair and refused to get out of it. While he rocked faster and faster, she got behind him as he rocked forward and pushed the chair, tipping him out of it, and then she triumphantly ran around and seated herself in it. From the expression on her face and the story she was telling, I was convinced that she was, in her mind, actually reliving the incident.

Then I regressed her further, back to two days prior to her birth. In obvious anguish and gasping for breath, she cried out, "Oh, it is so heavy. There is too much pressure!" Tears streamed down her face, and her battle to breathe was so genuine that I put her back to sleep, brought her slowly forward through time and awakened her.

Evie was born the morning of March 12, 1954, at St. Francis Hospital in Miami Beach, Florida. Labor commenced about midnight and at 5:00 A.M., Dr. Salvatore Certo, attending obstetrician, informed her father that his child would be born shortly. She finally arrived about 9:00 A.M., after four hours of Herculean effort by Dr. Certo and his staff. The infant was completely enmeshed in the umbilical cord, making normal delivery impossible, a fact that was discovered too late for a Caesarian section.

After our first hypnotic experiment, Evie decided she would like to relive her birth, remembering her feelings and impressions of it. I agreed, but decided as the birth effort was so terribly traumatic, to have her view her birth as an observer as opposed to actually experiencing it.

Placing her in a trance, I instructed her to look on the baby that would be Evie Rieder, in the womb and five months developed. Then I told her to look down and tell me everything she saw.

Slowly she started, "The child is purple—and kicking." I asked, "Why is she purple?"

Evie answered, "She is purple because she is struggling against the tube. She is kicking and she is—ugh—she does not like it at ALL—she does not like it!"

She was becoming upset so I admonished her, "Don't feel it; just see it; tell me what you see."

She continued, "It's a—pressure on her head. She is upside down; oh, it is very uncomfortable, not a pleasant thing. She has never been comfortable; it is very crowded, very pressured. The *tube* (umbilical cord) is wrapped—lord, you'd think they would make more room!"

Then I instructed her to tell me about the tube. She continued, "It is in her way, all around her stomach and her head." Then her voice rose and she stated vehemently, "She is trying to push her arm out, but the cord is there; she is bound up in the cord."

In response to a question as to how the baby looked otherwise, she said, "Oh, yeah, she's fat in spite of the cord!"

She was then advanced to six months' development and asked what she saw. She informed me that she could see the baby's eyes clearly, that they looked good and that she was more comfortable now, that things had shifted and the baby had become used to conditions in the womb.

Advancing her on to seven months, I inquired if the baby was feeling better, and she replied, "Oh, it is getting tight; she is getting bigger; she's growing and her feet are moving, just her feet. She is backwards; it is like she is just sitting there."

"Where is the tube?" I inquired, and she answered, "The tube is *all over her*—it is stuck up in her face there—oh! (groan) she has her *arms* in front of her face to block the tube; she is protecting her face with her arms. The rest of the tube is down around behind; it does not look good."

We then went forward to the eight month, and she whispered, "Boy is she big—she is getting big. That tube is all around; it is down her back, draped—it is not around her neck yet; it is draped around her shoulders and her forehead."

I asked if it got that way by moving around, and she replied, "Yes she moved around, but there was not enough room, seems to be more cord than room, more cord than is reasonable."

"Is she looking good?"

"She is very big and healthy. She would have to be to be alive because otherwise she would be dead—shredded—because of the cord; it pushed her."

Taking her to the ninth month, I admonished her again to just view the proceedings, not to feel anything. She continued, "Pulsating—that child's head is going to blow up! That baby's going to die; she is going to blow up her head! The cord is everywhere—God, between her feet, legs...." Then, registering amazement, she added, "She is standing in the womb (whispering); the baby's just standing there in the womb; she is trying to be born."

I inquired, "Where is her head?" and she answered, "Up in the womb."

Then I asked, "Is it in the birth canal?" and she answered with a disparaging note, "No," and added, "The cord is by her feet, around her body, around her neck, around her back and shoulders and under her right arm. Her head is on top—(whispering to herself in disbelief) she is STANDING on the womb; she is starting to be born!"

Prodding her on I queried, "Now what is happening?" and she went on, "She has got her foot out—trying to step out."

Now an interesting change occurred, and she continued as though she were talking to the baby. "What-cha gonna do?" Laughingly, "She is trying to STEP out of the womb—can't go that way!" As though speaking firmly to the baby, "Supposed to go the other W-A-Y...." Then she observed, "The doctor is going to turn her around; she is supposed to come out the other way. She did not know that, otherwise she would have tried—it was not easy getting like THAT in the first place—that was a struggle in itself. She is going to come out somehow—but—the way the cord is, that would make it difficult. Being upside down, she could be hanging on the cord." Emitting a long sigh she added, "She doesn't want to be turned around; she wants to come feet first and the doctor won't let her."

She paused for a while, then gave a painful groan. "Oh, God, the cord is all over there. The doctor is pushing her in—he pushed her feet back in—aah." Then she jumped perceptibly and grabbed at her neck. "He pushed her feet and that tightened the cord; her legs were straight and he bent them back up and that tightened the cord around her neck."

Another long sign, "The baby just does not dig it—now her feet are inside, and it seems to be general confusion. Just a lot of panic there—she was already to come out. Panic, boy, they don't know what to do (whispering)—let her do it!

"Let her do what?" I asked.

Still whispering, "Just step out." When I asked her why the doctor would not let her be born feet first, she answered resignedly, "The mother would die, yes, the mother would die." As an afterthought she whispered, "She'd have no pity." Elaborating, she explained that the baby would have no pity on her mother in order to be born, adding, "It is her life; she wants to live."

I asked what they were doing now and she said, "They pushed her in—(indignantly) that doctor just PUSHED HER IN. He is still trying to get the cord—he knows now that it is a problem; everyone is well aware that it is a problem. Now they are going to push her around—she is purple and pulsating. The baby's struggling—she is fighting, drowning."

"Drowning?"

Sadly, "Just drowning, yes. No air—she is not getting any air—the cord—the doctor is pulling." She was becoming frantic, observing closely what was transpiring. "Once they get over THAT point it will be all right. He is trying to turn her ALL the way around, and once they get over that—and the cord is stuck—if they just make THAT point, it will be all right."

Then she spoke as though she were directing the doctor, "Just get her half way around, get the cord off her neck." Continuing to observe, "He has got to turn her all the way around to get the cord from around her neck; he is trying." Again she was becoming extremely agitated, and I cautioned her not to feel it, just to see it, to observe.

Another long sigh and she declared that the baby was almost turned, that they needed to pull her down a little more. Describing how the doctor had turned her, she stated that he had just put his hand up there and pushed her, and that the baby was fighting him.

Remembering that there had been two nurses and an intern pushing her from the outside, I inquired if she felt other pressure and she answered, "Yes, everywhere she goes there are people pushing her another way. They literally lifted her up, it seems like, and turned her over." Then she nodded her head reassuringly and said that the baby was now in position to be born.

When I asked what her mother was doing, Evie answered, "I don't know, but she is not digging it. Her mother is having problems. She does not know what to do, whether to hold back or let go—and the pain is bad. She is yelling now but she has not always been yelling. She is not screaming too bad—there has always been a lot of noise. The baby is turned around to the other side now; the cord is getting looser. When one loop is relaxed, then they can loosen it all around her body."

She explained that they were loosening the cord very carefully and that they did not understand it had been there a long time. She said the doctor was doing it with his hands and that it was painful for the baby but that she knew what he was doing and why. Then she made an observation that surprised me. She said, "The doctor could have made the difference."

"What do you mean?"

"Well, they could have been dead, the baby and the mother—but the doctor worked hard, everybody worked."

Describing the baby as still wrapped in the cord but able to be born, she said the doctor had his hand on her head, holding her back—she did not know why.

This was probably when they were giving me pure oxygen in an attempt to minimize any damage that may have occurred to the baby. This was followed immediately by gas and Dr. Certo performed an episiotomy (a cut in the vaginal orifice to facilitate the birth) and she was born. She described the actual birth as quick and said that they cut the cord in order to finish unwrapping it from her.

She jumped again after saying this and cried out that they had covered her face with an oxygen mask and made her breathe. It was cold and gave her an awful shock and she did not like it at all. Then she added that they were "waving her around" and slapping her rear end and that the baby did not care much for that either.

Smiling, I said to her, "Now they are laughing; they are laughing because you are a girl, and what did your mother desperately want?"

Evie gave me a radiant, illuminating smile and answered, "A girl. My mother wanted a girl. Everybody is happy; they are all excited and smiling."

I continued, "You are a fat, healthy baby and you are very happy to finally be in the world and to have the birth all behind you, aren't you?" She nodded in agreement and I went on, "They have cut the cord, put something in your eyes to protect them and now what are the nurses saying?"

She answered, "They are saying that the baby is cute; they are remarking how cute and fat she is."

Then I directed her to continue with the story, asking her what they were doing with her foot. She answered that they were wiggling it, putting something on her ankle and pressing her foot against something. This would be the footprint that is taken of all newly born babies and the item they put on her ankle would be the identification tag. She then described how they were fussing over her, and later she told me about seeing her father for the first time. Her words were, "He is very excited—oh, he is so happy—he likes me a lot. Now he is holding me—no, now they are taking me away, putting me back with all the babies." Then she added something I consider to be hilarious—under her breath she whispered, "Boring."

Evidently, after being the undivided center of everyone's attention for so long, she found being just another baby in the hospital nursery dull.

We decided, at a later date, to see just how far back in her development she could find awareness. It had always been my conception (or misconception) that a fetus became viable, or life started, at about five months' development. This is why I had previously picked the fifth month as a starting point. Consequently, we started our second experiment at the five-month point, only this time instead of coming forward, we would continue to regress for as long as there was perception.

At five months she reiterated that it was very cramped, crowded with a great deal of pressure. Back to four months and she described the baby as being "Right up against the wall, crowded, in a fetal position. She is at the top of the uterine wall, in the 2 o'clock position." She added that it was between four and five months that the cord started being a serious problem. At three months she said, "Flat, I feel flat and round. The eyes are developed, everything is developed, and the cord is around my left arm."

Back to two months and she described the fetus as very small, pretty well formed—hands and feet are partially formed, pointed. She is way up in the corner, in the top of the womb, "all squished up." Physical sensation is very limited. The brain is so big, and it feels encompassed, and again there is a feeling of roundness. Her memories are of almost everything, as though she were everything. She does not feel as though she is an individual, it is as though she were one with the universe. It is a weird feeling, she stated.

Evie described the fetus at one month as being about two or three inches big (holding up her fingers in a measuring gesture). She is there in the corner all curled up. Her mind is working but not with any exactness at all—not like before. She is just barely aware of being there and does not discern anything much—nothing matters much, but she is aware.

There was almost no consciousness at two weeks of development, just a constant hum that went on all the time. It was her life force, the pulsating blood. Later, when conscious, she said that the first two weeks were frantic. All one could hear was the hum of the blood flowing through one's veins and the cells reproducing at such a frantic rate that, if you were to think about it, you would probably be in pain. She was not aware of the cord at that time and felt it did not become a problem until much later. She felt that at five weeks there was a leveling off period and at that time the rapid cell division slowed down. It was at the point of five weeks that she felt that the baby started having awareness as an entity.

She said, "Those first five weeks are a hard time. I can see that if a fetus does not make it, it would most likely be at that time. A lot of them don't make it, I imagine. They just fall off (the uterine wall) and the woman does not even know she was pregnant.

While she was still hypnotized, I inquired if she could see the actual conception. After a wait, she said, "The awareness is—it's a little pinpoint of an egg—I can see it, there are other eggs. I feel an affinity to one. It gets PUNCTURED! (Pain in her voice) it's like a little fish; they are all over (the sperm cells). You can FEEL their thrust, their purpose. Pushing, it's crazy, lots of them are trying to puncture that egg but they bounce off. One of them manages to puncture the egg. It does not come into the egg, just it's head. Very painful—then things change, like the war is over."

She was not aware that the egg had moved, and said it was stationary when punctured, that it was on the uterine wall in the same place that the baby would grow.

In the conscious state, Evie described the conception process as being like "planned chaos." She recalled seeing the egg in the ovary with all the other little eggs. Laughing, she described it as being like a little race or game to see which one gets there first. "I had an awareness of my egg, but I did not know if that one was going to get inseminated. I had an awareness of other eggs, too, and I felt that, if another egg had become fertilized, I would have become a different person—the same, but different."

She said the actual conception was like a little war game and that, after the egg was punctured, it was like the calm after a storm. There was no feeling of consciousness connected to the sperm; it was as though it was just a servicing factor. "The consciousness is strictly in the egg," she stated and added, "the sperm is mindless, a driving, dynamic force."

As we concluded, she informed me that the questions I asked her when she was hypnotized were too specific. She said she felt as though she were one with the universe, an ethereal feeling impossible to explain. She considered it to be almost a religious experience and felt that prenatal influences help shape whatever religious convictions one has through life.

Also, she observed, time and the present are not important. One has a feeling of being tied to all the past and to all the future. Interestingly enough, she said that there is a feeling of indifference as to whether or not the egg does become fertilized, and if it does, whether or not it survives for the first three or four months.

After the forth month of development, the fetus is more like an unborn baby and is prepared to put up a fight for survival.

It is interesting to note that today Evie refuses to wear turtlenecked sweaters, bras, anything tight or constricting around her upper torso. Since this experiment was conducted, Evie has described it as the most profound experience of her life. It expanded her consciousness, she stated, and she views it as a sort of religious epiphany.

Prior to undertaking this study, I was firmly on the side of the abortionists, feeling that a woman has a right to make this sort of decision. Now I am very ambivalent in my feelings and am eternally grateful that this is one choice which I have never been forced to make!

Following is an interesting conclusion to this story. In 1950 when I gave birth to my son, the cord was around his neck three times. It did not, however, interfere with the birth. When I discussed this with the doctor, his reply was, "Don't give it another thought; it won't happen again in a million years." Dr. Certo, who delivered Evie, had said the same thing to me prior to her birth.

In December of 1985, my daughter-in-law gave girth to my first grandchild. My son called me from New York on November 27th to inform me that the baby would be delivered around December 1st by Caesarean section. When I inquired why a Caesarean, his answer was, "Because the sonar scope shows that the baby is breech and completely wound up in the cord!"

PLANNED CHAOS
by Evie Rieder

I was first—NO! I was too!
Who am I? and ... who are you?
Move aside ... NO! get together.
Will it be this way forever?
I moved once, you moved twice,
we kicked us, we're not nice.
Lennon said it all too well,
"Come together" from this cell.
Once there was one ... now two, perhaps three.
"I am you and you are me"
Transport time and move in place,
all of life wants in this race.
Eventually all will calm down,
won't be as much movement around.
I am night and I am day.
So it is ... God's fit that way.
No accidents or unplanned deeps,
I'm comfortable with what I see.
"Yes, we're in this thing together."
It WILL be that way forever!
I'll be black and I'll be white.
I'll be good and I'll be right.
Never understand the choice,
didn't recognize the voice.
Let it go and "Let it be."
We are exact ... perhaps ... maybe.

CHAPTER TEN

TWIN STUDY

WHILE WORKING ON MY MANUSCRIPT, "Truth Revealed by Time," it became increasingly evident to me that the "past lives" people relive and discuss while experiencing hypnotic regression might be, in some way, memories they have inherited.

The story of "Truth" is that of a young woman currently living in Anaheim, California. When hypnotized, she has given vivid details of the life of a queen born in Sweden in 1626.

During the course of the research, evidence surfaced that the queen, Christina, left a child in Hamburg, Germany, in the year 1666. Until now, history has been unaware of the possibility of this child.

The subject of the experiment is of German descent and, when I discovered that her mother's family seat in Germany was the small town of Kiel, located a few miles from Hamburg, there arose a suspicion that she had inherited this memory somehow—if not through genes per se, then perhaps through some other avenue of transmission. Even the possibility of a psychic link passed down through the generations has been suggested by some modern scientists.

At first I decided to try an ethnic test. That is to say, if I were to regress a great many people of "pure" ethnic origin, and they, while regressed, remained true to their ethnic background, then this might be indicative of inheritance of memory.

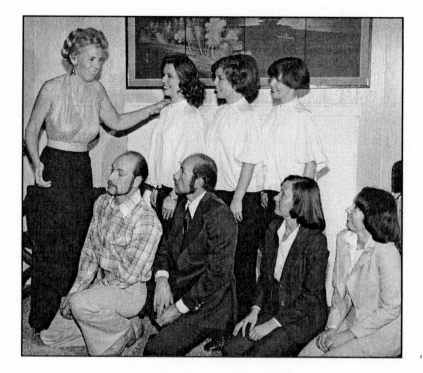

Twins and triplets used in the study
Photo by Bob Wheeler, *O.C. Register*

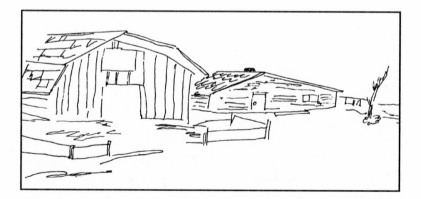

Sketch of farm in Wyoming or Montana done by Dave Morgan

However, when one considers that we all have two parents, four grandparents, eight great grandparents, and we continue to square with each generation back, true "ethnic purity" becomes highly questionable. Searching for another course, I decided that work with identical twins might be enlightening. Identical twins occur when the zygote, or fertilized egg, divides, producing the two fetuses each bearing a chromosome and genetic pattern identical to the other. If my theory regarding inherited memory is correct, that is, that the "past lives" people live under hypnotic regression is in fact a memory passed down through the generations, then identical twins, who share the same genes and physical structure, should share the same memories.

It was my experience that they do!

The first set of twins I regressed were Doris and Debbie Ball, both residents of Orange County, California. The girls were twenty-nine years of age, average height, slender with dark hair and eyes, very light skin and exceptionally attractive. Doris was a mobile home saleswoman, and Debbie teaches school on the college level.

Doris was interviewed first, apart from her sister. Instructing her to regress to the year 1760, I told her to go to the age of twenty in that lifetime. Her description was that she had long brown hair, blue eyes, was of medium height and slender. She was not married but had a lot of friends, she related. Taking her ahead to age twenty-five, she said that now she was married to a very nice man. He was tall with dark hair and was always dressed up in a suit. He worked in town in a bank, she said, made a lot of money and took good care of her. At age thirty in the same life she said that she had two children, a boy and a girl. At age sixty she described the woman as being semi-invalid in a beautiful bedroom with a "big, fluffy bed made of beautiful wood." Also in the bedroom was a dresser with a large mirror. A uniformed maid was caring for her, and she ate off a tray with a silver cover over the food.

Taking her further back, we regressed her to the year 1600. She said she was on a BIG sailing ship and had been on it for a long time.

Her description of herself was that she was a female with long yellow hair, blue eyes and pretty. She explained that her folks were sending her to England to attend boarding school to get her away from a young man they considered unsuitable for her. Her age she gave as about seventeen. Going back to the thirteenth year, she described a scene wherein her family and some of their relatives were barricaded in a house. There were a lot of people outside with guns, threatening and shooting at them. her father fired back and the people left. Later some friends had come and taken them all away, out into the country and to safety.

Going back much further, still in the same lifetime, she described a scene that caused her to exhibit a lot of emotion. Obviously she was viewing something that frightened her. She described herself as a little girl about four or five years old. She was hiding at the base of a large tree, watching a large group of men. They wore black capes and tall black hats and were up to no good, she stated. There was a man on the ground with his feet bound and they were yelling and threatening him. The girl was frightened because she was not supposed to be there. She said that one of the men had a gun and another a rope in a circle (coiled). When I asked her what the men were doing, she put her hands over her face and cried (while peeking between her fingers), "I am not watching!"

The study with twins denoted one fact quite clearly. Of a set of twins, one is usually more extroverted and intrepid than the other. The extrovert will tell the story with more embellishment, and take less coaxing and probing than with the more introverted twin.

When I hypnotized Debbie, it was immediately obvious that she was the more audacious of the two. Her answers and descriptions were firm and unhesitating. Her story was essentially the same as Doris'. We regressed to the year 1760 and suggested she go to age twenty. She described herself exactly as her sister had: unmarried, long brown hair, blue eyes, etc. At age twenty-five she stated she was married to a tall, handsome man who had a lot of money and worked in a ... bank? At age thirty she was very happy and had two children, a boy and a girl. Advanced to age sixty she gave the same description her sister had of a bedroom with a large four-poster bed, a tall dresser with a mirror and water pitcher; the furniture was made of a beautiful wood, probably oak.

Going back to the year 1600 she told of being on a ship for a long, long time, and her description of herself jives with the one her sister had given for that period of time—light yellow hair, blue eyes, not fat. She explained that she was going to boarding school and she was not happy about it—she missed the boy she loved and was forced to leave. She was more emphatic than her sister about the unhappiness the girl on the ship was experiencing.

Her story when she was a teenager and the house was under siege matched that of her sister. She related how angry the people surrounding the house were and how frightened she and her parents became, adding that she was hiding under the bed and her father was shooting at the intruders and that her mother had been slightly wounded in the melee. She also told how friends came and rescued the family.

Directing her to go back to the time that the little girl was watching the men in the black capes and hats, she described how the little girl hid behind the base of a large tree and how frightened she was of being discovered, explaining that the men had instructed her to go home. Then she volunteered the information that they were *hanging* that man from a tree and that the little girl did not understand what was happening.

The second set of twins to cooperate with me in my study were Dan and Dave Morgan from Riverside, California. The men were thirty-one years old, of average height and build with sandy colored hair and blue eyes. Their father is full-blooded Italian and their mother is of French-English heritage.

Because the Ball girls are what hypnotists call "instant somnambulists," they were able to enter the trance state very quickly and in only two comparatively short sessions I was able to obtain their story. However, the Morgan twins were of an entirely different makeup and required a great deal more time and work on my part in order to get them into a regressable trance state.

Hypnosis is generally described as an altered state of consciousness. A person's brain wave pattern changes under hypnosis,
differing from the pattern emitted during the sleeping and waking
states. This denotes that a physiological change or changes occur to
a person undergoing hypnosis—physiological reactions to a psychological stimulus.

Normally, responses to identical words presented in the same
manner by the same person will have a wide variance from one
person to another. This statement is definitely not true of identical,
single-egg persons, at least as far as hypnosis is concerned. With
the twins and later on the triplets, their responses became entirely
predictable. Each twin or triplet would follow the exact hypnotic
pattern of their siblings. The Ball twins required only two easy
sessions to tell their story, while the Morgan twins each started to
regress late in the third meeting, and the triplets each required five
lengthy meetings before becoming regressable. I became completely familiar with the fleeting little self-conscious smile that
played around the lips of all three of the Brown triplets at the advent
of their first two sessions. Having observed it during my work with
the first one, it did not surprise me when the other two adhered to
the identical pattern at the same stage in the induction. This might
indicate that a great many more of our responses are prepro-
grammed than the Freudian school of psychology is wont to
acknowledge.

Each of the Morgan twins, when regressed, described a man
they saw living in a jungle. He lived in a hut made of bamboo
covered with large leaves. There were monkeys playing nearby and
the man was wearing torn and tattered clothes.

Dave said he felt that the man had been deserted there as a
young man and had made friends with the black natives. In his old
age they both pictured him with a long gray beard and very dark
skin, from the sun. They natives, they both said, had taken care of
the old man in his later years.

Both boys were able to go strongly into character in the role of
a young farmer who had a farm in the high country of either

Montana or Wyoming. Each described the mountains in the distance and the high pine trees that surrounded the clearing where the farm was located. The barn, they both agreed, was near the house and there was a watering trough near the gate by the road. When I asked Dan who was the president of the country, he answered, "I want to say Teddy Roosevelt."

After Dave awakened from the trance, he sketched for me the layout of the farm—the house, barn and fence. Later when Dan became conscious after describing the same scene, I showed him the picture his brother had drawn and he immediately identified it as what he had seen, explaining that Dave had viewed it from a different angle than he had when seeing it.

One thing I noticed about the boys was that immediately prior to becoming regressed, they both complained that their legs ached and that they had an overpowering urge to bring their knees up to their chest. At first I thought this had something to do with the personality they were regressing to, but as both described different life times to me after announcing this desire to raise their legs, I can only assume that immediately before regressing they both experienced a return to the womb motivation, a desire to assume the fetal position.

Realizing that three of a kind always beats a pair, I was delighted when the Brown triplets volunteered to help me in my experiment.

According to the girls, they became triplets when the fertilized egg their mother produced divided in half and then one half redivided. The doctor that delivered them ascertained that Pamela, the first-born, developed from the half egg, and Peggy and Patrice resulted from each quarter egg.

The Brown triplets were the only set of identical triplets born anywhere in the world in the year 1952. They were raised in Santa Ana, California, and Pamela and Peggy still reside in Orange County, while Patrice currently lives in Arizona.

The girls are short and petite in stature, have brown hair and brown eyes, and exquisitely flawless English-style complexions.

They are perky, vivacious, extremely loquacious and proved to be difficult to hypnotize. Their father is of English descent and their mother is an interesting combination of English, Spanish and American Indian.

Several weeks were spent working alternately with Pamela and Peggy; then I traveled to Arizona to regress Patrice. The stories of all three girls were essentially similar with one glaring exception which I will describe later.

All three of the girls described a beautiful English girl with brown hair, blue eyes and an exceptionally lovely complexion and features. When instructed to go into the morning of her twentieth birthday, they all saw a canopied bed with a beautiful satin coverlet which Pamela described as white, and Peggy saw as pink or white. Patrice was unsure of the color but insisted it was very light. Each one agreed there was a very ornate gold mirror on the wall and each identified a uniformed maid that entered the girl's room on that morning. I suggested that they move from the bedroom into the hall; they individually described a hall with plush reddish carpet containing a gold design. Peggy and Patrice elaborated that the carpet design was of an acorn shape or motif. There were tables against the wall, they said, and a wide, massive staircase leading down to the first floor with a large chandelier overhead. Pamela and Peggy both saw a painting of the girl on a wall at age seven or eight. The little girl was posed sitting on a large chair, and both of them mentioned that something about the portrait reminded them of the famous painting of "Pinky" by Gainsborough.

Going to another lifetime or memory, all three of them told of seeing a young girl with flamboyantly red hair. Peggy described her hair as "orange," and Patrice said it was "carrot-red." Pamela claimed that the youngster was homely, Patrice said she was pretty ugly, and Peggy exclaimed, "Lord, what an ugly kid!" They saw her as living in poverty in her early years, wearing ratty, raggedy clothes. Advancing to the girl's late twenties, Patrice was unable to see her, but Pamela and Peggy both used the same words to remark that they saw the girl as having "moved up in the world." They both said she had married a man with money, and they both saw her dressed very elegantly.

One personality they all three saw very clearly and were in complete accord on was the life of a young girl that they felt was English who had a deep love of horses and was an accomplished equestrian. They all pictured her as wearing a riding outfit. The girl was not exceptionally beautiful but was very attractive. She had warm brown hair which she tied in the back, and she wore a hat with her riding habit.

Peggy and Pamela both described an English manor house with French-type windows divided into little squares. The entrance hall of the house contained a large table where she laid her hat and crop. There was a very straight staircase near the hall with highly polished steps, white posts and a gleaming, lacquered handrail.

Patrice saw her at a later time, when she was married and living in a colonial-style home. All three portrayed the arena where she exercised her horse when she was young as circular and bordered by a white picket fence. They said she rode almost daily down a path through a woods, and all saw a typical hunting dog running alongside the horse. Descriptions of the dog were identical. They saw it as small, black and white and golden tan with a long tail and medium length ears. All three saw her winning many cups and ribbons in riding competitions, and Peggy and Patrice agreed that she married very well, Peggy claiming she married a statesman and Patrice stating that the husband had an important position, like an attorney or maybe in government.

During her last really deep regression Pamela mentioned a "chair or white throne?"—very ornate, with a lot of gold trim and a velvet cushion. Peggy described the chair as possibly being the throne of a royal personage. It was white, she declared, with a great deal of gold on it. It was very petite appearing and was decorated with scrolling. All the girls described the arms of the chair as circling out from the back, and Patrice emphasized that the chair was heavily decorated with very ornate carving or scrolling.

Pamela pictured to me a room in a house, very old, with a cobblestone-type floor. Old pots and pans were hanging around the walls and the furniture was very sparse and rough. There was a rugged old wooden chair and a long, plain wooden table supporting a coffin—a plain wooden coffin with black metal work. She was standing in the room viewing the coffin and was aware of a *distraction* between herself and the coffin, not moving but stationary. She could not ascertain what the distraction was. Peggy, when I directed her to see the room that contained the coffin, reaffirmed that it was a very old house, "really ugly—much poverty." She added that the house was very dingy and dirty and musty. Then, before I could question her regarding the distraction Pamela had seen, she declared, "There is a RAT on the floor. He is against the wall, just standing there—stationary—and staring at me with his beady little eyes!"

She described herself as an older woman wearing a black dress with a white apron in the front. Patrice collaborated the description of the room and the coffin and added that there was a stone fireplace in the room that looked as though it had been used a lot. She was unaware of the rat and described herself as a woman wearing a dark dress and a bonnet.

The most intriguing story the girls gave me was that of an Hawaiian girl. They portrayed her as average height, brown eyes, long brown hair and very pretty. Pamela and Peggy pictured her as living in a shack-type of place on the beach near the ocean with palm trees between the shack and the water. The girl's bed was a cot-like affair, very simple and looked homemade. They described the happy, carefree life that the island girl lived.

Each one of the triplets had the same reaction to questions about the girl's mother. Their faces lit up and a very amused expression surfaced. Each one described the mother as being very heavy, short and a jovial type person. Peggy volunteered, "She has a great laugh!" When I quizzed Patrice about the mother's laugh, she beamed and agreed, "Oh, yes!"

Now comes the glaring discrepancy in the regression stories of the triplets.

Pamela described the Hawaiian girl's wedding as taking place outdoors. She could hear water out in front, either a stream or a fountain. There were a lot of people present, but it was not a huge group.

She saw the groom as wearing white, with a lei of flowers around his neck. She was uncertain if what he was wearing was a uniform or a service suit of some type. The feast that was to follow was being prepared; there was a pig, buried. Several men and women were doing a Hawaiian dance similar to the hula, and there was a large drum, like a big barrel and looking like a bongo drum.

Then she stated that the man she had married had a light skin, medium brown hair and was good looking. He was thin and rather slight of build. He was definitely a Caucasian and she thought he was English. They had three or four children, beautiful children that were all much lighter than their mother. None of them were twins.

Imagine my shock when Peggy described the husband of the Hawaiian girl as "really tall, he is wearing a lei and a skirt or shorts—it is a skirt outfit (lava-lava) that Hawaiians wear, very colorful. He has real dark hair with dark eyebrows and a little bit of hair on his chest. He is Hawaiian; he is like—the king's son, I guess."

I inquired if she saw a man in a white suit, and her answer was that there was a man in a white suit and hat who had a Bible in his hand and that he was definitely not the groom, that he was either a missionary or a preacher. There were two pigs roasting in the ground, and she claimed that the wedding was huge. Giggling, she confided that the girl was very much in love and could hardly wait for the honeymoon to commence. Her big preoccupation with the wedding other than the groom was the girl's wedding dress—it was white and Hawaiian in design. She stated that she could hear Hawaiian music, a guitar and several drums. The feast was commencing, and she again described the entire ceremony as "just huge."

Going ahead in time she said the girl had two boys and a little girl. They were all dark, but not as dark as their father. I asked her if the girl may have been widowed and later married an American or Englishman and received a positive, "No!"

The blatant discrepancy in the stories Pamela and Peggy told about the Hawaiian girl had me extremely puzzled, but I suspected what the answer might be.

Describing the girl's wedding, Patrice claimed that the girl's dress was long and flowery, with colors of green and blue. There was a halo of flowers in her hair and a lot of people—the ceremony was taking place outside. Then she said the groom was tall with dark hair and very good looking, and definitely Hawaiian. Then she declared he was wearing a white outfit—"not a suit, but a white jacket and white pants." Later she saw the girl with probably three children, two of whom were pretty close—"boys" and she thought they were born together, "twins." At that time I instructed her to take the Hawaiian girl back into her mother's womb, just prior to her birth. She stated that she saw two babies, that the Hawaiian girl had had a twin sister.

My suspicions were confirmed. The Hawaiian girl had been twins, and Pamela had inherited the memory of one twin and Peggy the other. It would appear that Patrice had received a composite of the two memories, at least as far as the wedding was concerned, as she pictured the husband of one girl as the groom of the other.

This revelation exposes another area of thought and speculation. Could the extrapolation of the memory genes be lateral as well as longitudinal? Is it possible that when genes divide, as in the case of identical twins or triplets, that during the years that follow, as the memory travels from generation to generation, the gene has a tendency to recombine or become whole again, causing the memory of twins to converge, giving the recipient the memory of a single entity instead of a multiple birth?

Another question that surfaces is whether it could be that the factor that triggers a fertilized egg to divide may travel in these memory genes, meaning that all identical twins and triplets have, somewhere deep in their minds, memories of other lifetimes when they lived as part of a multiple birth?

In this study, the participants were hypnotized individually. Much earlier, while I was attending school, an experiment was undertaken with two young girls about eighteen years old. They were hypnotized together and taken back into a past life, and it was an extremely amusing session.

As they both experienced the same past life, they would argue and bicker about what they were seeing. One twin would say, "She was wearing her new shoes," and the other would retort, "No, she didn't wear them that day," and her sister would agree, "That's right, her mother said they had to be fixed."

CHAPTER ELEVEN

PHANTOM LIMB PAIN

In my early days as a hypnotist, a young man came to see me. He was about twenty-five years old, average size, and his left arm was missing from just above the elbow.

As we talked, the stump of his left arm jumped and twitched, always in motion.

He explained to me that he had been in the Army, stationed in Germany, when there had been a motorcycle accident resulting in the loss of his arm. The accident had occurred about three years earlier, and he had experienced excruciating pain in the missing arm intermittently since its amputation. One of the last things the Army doctor told him regarding the phantom limb pain was "See a hypnotist."

Being very candid with him, I explained this was the first case of phantom limb pain I had ever seen, and of course, I had never worked with anyone to allay it. However, I told him, I was more than willing to try.

He was a good subject and went into a trance very easily.

My suggestions were that he could see into his brain. There were nerves there, something like electrical circuits, and he could find the ones leading down into the missing arm. "What position are those nerves in," I asked him, "the ON or OFF position?"

His answer was, as I expected, that the nerves were in the ON position.

"Now you are pulling the lever that controls the nerves leading to your missing arm into the OFF position. You are pulling the lever firmly down. To make certain it stays down, you are firmly tying it down with some excess tissue you find there. Now there is no longer any sensation of any type in the missing arm."

The suggestions worked like a charm, and the young man had no more pain. He called me the following week and said he had had the first night's sleep, after I hypnotized him, that he had had since the accident.

Since that experience, I have worked, successfully I might add, with several persons suffering from phantom limb pain.

A few years ago, when I moved into the mobile home park in which I now reside, I was invited to a Christmas party. There I met a most charming woman. As we talked, she pointed out to me her husband across the room. "He's such a dear man," she exclaimed, "and he suffers so terribly."

Seems he is diabetic and had a leg amputated just below the knee. For seven years he had bouts of severe pain. "Sometimes he suffers so much he sits on the living room floor and cries and massages the stump of his leg," she further stated.

Mentioning that I am a hypnotist, I suggested that I most likely could help him.

The next morning I went to their coach. Walt was there alone. Because he is such a gentleman, he agreed to be hypnotized, all the while informing me that it would not work. He had been hypnotized for smoking and that had not worked, and besides, he could not be hypnotized. As I said, Walt is the ultimate gentleman, and he probably thought it would be rude not to humor me.

While placing him quickly into a deep trance, I suggested that his right hand would become very light and lift slowly up off of his lap. When the hand was pointing towards the ceiling, I gave him the suggestions concerning turning off the errant nerves in his brain. Then I touched his hand lightly with orders that it drop back into his lap, which it immediately did.

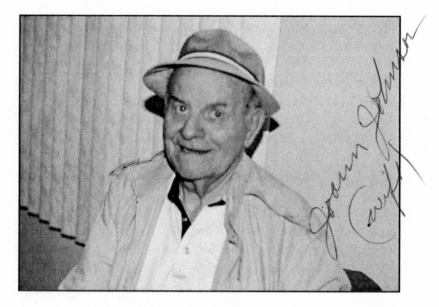

Walt Johnson, free of pain

He awoke laughing. "Boy, you had me under," he said in amazement. "I was lying there, listening to what you were saying when all of a sudden I felt my hand go 'plop' into my lap, and I thought to myself, I'll be damned, she's got me hypnotized." Then he shook his head in utter amazement; opening his eyes wide, he stared at me. "By George, the pain is gone. I feel nothing, no pain, no sensation of any kind. Glory be, the pain is gone!" I had a believer!

Several months later, Walt's wife called me to say that Walt was suffering from an unidentifiable pain in his stomach and could I help. My answer was that I could do nothing until he had been cleared by a doctor. It seems he had been hospitalized for six days, undergone every test known to modern medicine to no avail. The doctors could find nothing wrong with him.

Arriving at his home, I discovered his two granddaughters were with him. They asked if they could watch and I agreed.

He was in a deep trance and I was discussing the pain with him when one of the girls passed a note to me asking that I regress him into a past life. This I did, suggesting that he regress to a lifetime wherein he had suffered a similar abdominal pain.

He was a lieutenant in the Confederate Army, I was told, and General Lee had just finished chewing him out because his uniform was dirty. He was from a wealthy family in Baton Rouge, Louisiana, and planned to go into the family import business after the war.

I asked if the young man had survived the war and heard, "No, he was killed in a skirmish a few months before the war ended."

"Was he shot?" I inquired.

"No, he was bayoneted in the gut. He died very quickly."

The Lieutenant was told to be aware of the bayonet, the pain, and as the weapon was pulled from his body, he bled to death within a few minutes. Then I brought Walt up to the present time and out of the trance.

He smiled at me and said, "When you described that Yank pulling the bayonet out of my stomach, the pain went right out with it. There is no more pain at all!"

The last time I helped Walt with pain, it was because he had received a new prosthesis which failed to fit properly. It had caused an angry abrasion on the stump of his leg.

This time I tried something different—something called "glove anesthesia." I suggested to him that his right hand was completely numb. To check I pricked his hand with a pin. When there was no response, I knew his hand was feelingless. Then I directed him to sit up and place the numb hand directly onto the painful stump. When he had done this, I stated that the numbness would transfer from his hand into the area under the hand. When he could feel his hand again, he could remove it, and the stump would be numb and have no feeling or sensation. The numbness would last, I continued, until he could get his new prosthesis fixed, and until that time he would wear his old one. Then I told him to take a short nap.

About ten minutes later, as I sat in the kitchen having a cup of coffee with his wife, Walt, wearing his old leg and a big smile, walked into the kitchen and inquired, "Any chance of getting some lunch around here?" From this I could assume he was no longer in pain.

A couple of years after I had first worked with Walt Johnson, I received a call from a young man who lived in Wisconsin. He had heard about my work with Walt from one of Walt's relatives and asked if he could come to see me. He arrived a few days later. His arm had been amputated between the shoulder and elbow a few years earlier, the result of injuries sustained in an automobile accident. The pain had become intolerable, to the point where he was suicidal. Several surgeries had been performed upon him, all unsuccessful. In the latest, doctors had cut nerves in his back in an effort to alleviate the pain. Dr. William Kroger has stated in his books that controlling pain by suggestion in phantom limb cases is much more difficult if the patient has been subjected to surgery to treat that pain. I found this to be very true.

My first session with the man from Wisconsin was only partially successful. He felt a definite diminishing of pain after the first treatment, but the pain was definitely still there.

The next morning I tried something that had only recently occurred to me. It is based on work that I had seen reported on television. The research was conducted by Dr. Thelma Moss and her associates at U.C.L.A., involving Kirlian photography. Kirlian (named for Russian researchers Semyon and Valentina Kirlian) photography is a highly sophisticated type of photography, requiring specialized equipment that photographs the corona discharge, or aura, from an object. One of the more interesting results of Kirlian photography is the phantom leaf phenomenon. This occurs when, after a whole leaf is photographed, a section of the leaf is cut away. When the mutilated leaf is rephotographed, occasionally the corona or aura assumes that of the original leaf—the light and outline continues on around where the original leaf outline had been. This phenomenon occurs only occasionally.

Utilizing this theory, I put the man into a trance and instructed him to see himself from above, as if he were up on the ceiling peering down. Then I suggested he see himself, his whole body, as it had been prior to the accident. He was to be very aware of the body's aura, the glow emitted from the electromagnetic discharge. He was able to see the intact body and its corona.

Then I instructed him to see the body after the accident: Describe the body's aura. Where is it in relation to the missing arm? The corona, he stated, was still traveling around the body as if it were intact. The aura shone and glimmered around the area where the *arm was gone!*

Taking my cue, I said, "I am now taking hold of the aura, about seven inches below the stump of your arm. I have a pair of special shears. I am severing the aura from the other side of the stump, and I am bending the seven inches of aura under the bottom of the stump, and I am blending it into the corona on the other side. I have cut away the aura from the missing section of arm. Now your body is totally intact, and the aura around the missing arm is now also missing.

When the young man awoke from the trance with a huge grin on his face, I was delighted. It was the first time I had seen him smile. His entire demeanor changed. When he arrived at my door, he was nervous, high strung and in pain, tension exuding from every pore. When he left, he was smiling, relaxed and excited. Excited only, he told me, because he had just received his life back!

CHAPTER TWELVE

SPIRIT RELEASEMENT

WHEN I FIRST READ AN ARTICLE by William Baldwin, D.D.S., Ph.D., in the *Journal of Regression Therapy,* published by A.P.R.T. (Association for Past-life Research and Therapy), concerning spirit releasement therapy, my reaction was, strangely enough, one of extreme anger. I thought to myself, "What is this? What idiotic nonsense is this man, with these advanced education credentials, writing about?"

The ancient concept of spirit possession, considered by many cultures to be valid, has been generally ignored by our modern-day society.

In former times the treatment of spirit possession was called exorcism, which any of us who saw the movie of that name will remember. Removal of malevolent or unfriendly spirits years ago was performed primarily by priests, usually Catholics and some-times medicine men or shamans.

After my initial reaction of anger abated, I studied more about the art and realized, to my astonishment, that it could work. Who cares what society's reaction might be to such a concept? If it works, makes people feel better, helps them abstain from aberrant behavior, and generally helps straighten out lives, then who cares?

Baldwin, in his article, states that modern methods of spirit releasement can bring profound and often unexpected results. I failed to realize how very true this statement was until I started practicing spirit releasement on some of my clients.

The presumption on which spirit releasement is based is that a discarnate spirit entity, the surviving personality or consciousness of a deceased human, can and sometimes does invade the psyche of a living person and influence the emotions, mental and physical functioning, and behavior of that person—generally in a negative way, particularly in the case of drug and alcohol addicts.

In some cases the possessing spirit may be that of an acquaintance, deceased friend or relative of the victim. More often, however, it is that of a total stranger, sometimes one who has died long before the lifetime of the possessed person.

As to why discarnate entities stage a parasitic takeover of the psyche of the victim, one can only speculate. Reasons for remaining on the earth plane given by the attaching spirits can be many and varied. Yes, we usually do discourse directly with the spirit. Those who are adversely affecting drug addicts had such a strong addiction to drugs in their own lifetime that they are loathe to give it up. Some are unaware of their death. They are thoroughly confused and find it easier to "hide" in their host than to make their own way to the next plane. Others are simply afraid to let go and prefer to hang on to a living person than face the unknown.

Attachment to a person may be random or accidental, or it can occur because of a physical proximity to the dying person at the time of their death. According to those, like Baldwin, who have studied the phenomenon extensively, nurses, doctors, policemen, medics or anyone close to a person at their time of death becomes a potential target.

There appears to be a variety of opinions as to what causes vulnerability to spirit attachment. Severe stress may open avenues to intrusion. Likewise use of alcohol or drugs may lower barriers. Surgery and anesthetic drugs used at the time may lower resistance and allow spirit entry.

Even though the victim is consciously unaware of attached spirits, the person's life can and will be strongly influenced in many ways by them. They very likely will exacerbate the intensity of emotions such as fear, anger, etc., often leading to inappropriate abreaction to many life situations.

The influences exerted by attached spirits can range from a minor energy drain to a major degree of interference in the host's life.

Logically, the goal of SRT (spirit releasement therapy) is to rid the victim of the invasive spirit. Sometimes PLT (past-life therapy) is involved because occasionally the parasitic entity dates back to a previous lifetime.

More often than not, the spirit is in no hurry to leave. The same reason that is keeping the spirit earthbound generally motivates them to remain, comfortably lodged in the host.

The initial step is to identify the spirit. Sometimes this is easy, sometimes not. Bear in mind the spirit has no wish or plan to leave. They will become evasive, argue or flatly refuse to leave.

The next step is to diagnose the type of spirit we are dealing with. Earthbound spirits of deceased humans are the most common and the easiest to deal with. It should be noted that there are other types of non-human and non-physical spirits that affect our lives. Here we are dealing with earthbound human spirits.

At this point, we attempt to engage the spirit in dialogue to discover why it chose to remain earthbound. Sometimes the spirit will become very angry; he or she will lie and eventually become downright abusive and nasty. At this point, the therapist must persevere—coaxing, cajoling, demanding that the spirit leave. The most effective method I have found, and one advocated by Dr. Baldwin, is to lead the conversation to a discussion of some- one, now deceased, that the spirit loved dearly, usually a close relative. One dwells on the revered one's attributes and lovability, usually resulting in a softening of attitude on the part of the spirit. Then the spirit is directed to gaze intently into a bright light on the horizon. In that light he sees the image of the loved one very clearly. The loved one is sometimes crying from loneliness and extending his or her arms to the spirit, pleading with the spirit to join the loved one in the light. Sometimes it takes a lot of arguing, insisting, coaxing and prodding to make this happen, but eventually it usually does.

During the latter part of this last stage, the hypnotized subject may behave erratically and in strange ways. Tears are most common, and I have witnessed severe physical convulsions and other types of abreactions.

The final step is to "seal up" the client. He or she is told to imagine a brilliant light starting in the solar plexus and extending out beyond the body. It forms a protective bubble of light surrounding the person, through which no spirit can enter.

After the spirit is released, the emotional state of the client usually continues, sometimes for hours. The overriding sentiment generally is elation and extreme gratitude that the disruptive spirit is gone.

This sort of therapy is especially effective when practiced upon alcoholic and drug-addicted persons.

Over the years I have done several spirit releasement procedures with various people, always with very dramatic results. Following are outlines of a few of those sessions.

The first person with whom I worked with spirit releasement was my daughter, Evie. The first entity to appear was a man named Thomas.

Thomas died in the early 1900s. Living in upstate Michigan, he was killed in a car accident and, after residing in other persons, attached himself to Evie when she was seven. Aged twenty-two when he died, Thomas had been a party boy whose parents had money. He was attending the University of Michigan at Ann Arbor, studying architecture, when he was killed, and has been on the earth plane since the accident. Remaining on earth was his decision, as he decided he was not good enough to leave. He was urging

Evie to self-destruct, and if she did, he would fasten himself to another entity. He felt strongly connected to this life even though it was not very rewarding.

"I hated my parents," Thomas stated, but he did love his grandmother, Nanny. He had one younger sister, and his opinion of her was, "She was a poof!"

Thomas was told that Nanny is "up in the light, waiting for you. She is terribly upset and lonely, and she has been waiting for you a long time."

"Can she bring me there?" he asked, and we assured him she could, and we would help him go to her. "Are you ready to go see Nanny?" I asked him, and he said he was. "You see the spirit of your Nanny; she is waiting for you; she will welcome and love you."

He answered, "She has her arms out toward me."

"You are helping Evie to heal," I told him. "As you leave Evie, you are allowing her to heal." I told him that we were traveling now and that he could see Nanny clearly, and she had her arms open to him. "How does she look?" I inquired, and he answered, "She looks wonderful; she is smiling now; she is happy; she is urging me to come."

While this discourse was transpiring, I had hold of his hand and was pulling his outstretched arm towards me. Suddenly he jumped slightly and pulled back. "I am so afraid," he cried. "Don't be afraid," I comforted him, "We are all with you. I am next to you; Evie's next to you; we are going to accompany you to Nanny. Keep your eyes focused on Nanny. Now she is smiling a beautiful smile. You are the only one who can make her smile like that, Thomas. Keep moving toward her; you continue to travel toward the light, and I want you to tell me when you are next to Nanny."

He answered, "Now I am next to Nanny."

"Now she is putting her arms around you, and she is hugging you. She is taking away all the pain, and she is giving you gladness.

You are very happy. Now you are where you belong, and it takes some getting used to, but you will remember that Nanny is right there all the time, Thomas. You are leaving now; you are leaving Evie to heal, and you are healing (throughout all this Evie was visibly shaking). For the first time in a long time you are feeling so good and so comfortable. You are completely encased in love, enclosed in Nanny's arms, and you are feeling the rapture and joy you did when you were a little boy." He agreed that it was wonderful to be so happy again; he did not think he could ever be this happy; it was a miracle. I closed the discourse with "You are up with Nanny now; you are completely gone from Evie and you are very happy!"

Then I instructed Evie to see a brilliant light in her body, near her solar plexus, and I touched the area below her breastbone. "Watch the light as it grows, glowing very strongly, and it keeps on growing, expanding to fill your entire body and completely fill the void that Thomas left. It continues to expand beyond Evie's body, all the way around; her entire body is surrounded by that light; it forms a protective, shimmering bubble of light. It is very strong and will protect you from any subversive influences. From time to time you will check on this light: close your eyes and make sure the bubble is intact, and if it is not, you will repair it. Any other spirits within you may leave through the skin of the bubble, but nothing can enter from the outside."

Another spirit that had invaded Evie was named Margarite. She was Spanish, lived in Guadalupe. Margarite was shot when she was thirty-two years old. Bandits raided her village in the 1930s, terrorizing the people and shooting indiscriminately. The unfortunate Margarite was a victim; she died immediately.

Because she had been a prostitute, Margarite had refused to leave the earth plane. Feeling she was impure, she refused to leave, attaching herself to Evie when Evie was about three. She was not happy with the situation but felt powerless to change it.

I explained to her that she had been shot and killed acciden-tally—it was not her fault—and that she had been a prostitute because it was the only way she could survive, that it was not a life she would have chosen, but there had been no alternative. "God has forgiven you," I continued, "now you must forgive yourself." It was pointed out to her that she had been forced into that lifestyle; it was a learning process for her soul.

Margarite admitted that the love of her life had been Joeseppi, her husband, who was now dead.

She was admonished to look into the light and see Joeseppi, which she did. "He is holding out his arms to me, saying come to me, my darling. He says he has been waiting a long time, *andale* (hurry). I want to go to him, but I am afraid."

She was reassured that we would accompany her on her voyage. "Hold out your hand to him, Margarite; see him take it. Watch him lead you out of this life plane, out of Evie; say good-bye to Evie. You don't need to be afraid." All this time Evie was shaking and sighing heavily.

Suddenly Evie announced that Margarite was gone. Though she was still shaking like a leaf, Evie stated that she was very happy, that she felt "lighter" and "cleaner." Then I gave her suggestions about placing the protective shield around her body and awakened her.

The next person I worked with was the son of a friend of mine. George (not his real name) was in his late twenties. He had several spirits disrupting him, but I will only describe one.

When George was in the trance, I announced that I wished to talk to one of the spirits.

I heard, in a firm voice, "This is Colby!" Colby announced that he was twenty when he died. "I got shot, about 1910, in New York City. Shot by one of the gendarme guys, a cop. I was having my fun strangling this broad...." He was getting very emotional. His par-ents had met at some sort of political rally expounding free love.

The rallies were held in a barn, and that is where he was conceived. He hated his mother, had absolutely no use for any woman, did not love anybody. "My mother was a whore; she was a bitch like every one of them!" He loved his dad, but his dad died when he was very young.

"Let's go back in time when you were with your dad, when you were very young." His face beamed and he looked very happy. Yes, he truly loved his father. I convinced him his father was waiting for him and would love and care for him.

It was not an easy chore. Colby had been a serial killer, George told me when he was conscious, and Colby was one mean, tough customer. Finally I was able to convince him to leave, but not until he had threatened me and every other woman who lived. His only joy in life, it appeared, was strangling women, primarily prostitutes.

After many minutes of coaxing and cajoling, Colby agreed to go with his father. George told me later that Colby was seriously considering attacking me while I was reasoning with him, but his great love for his father won out.

CHAPTER THIRTEEN

UTILIZING THE POWER OF THE UNCONSCIOUS MIND

SEVERAL YEARS AGO, I sold a ten-acre parcel of land. One morning, shortly after the escrow had closed, I was looking for the note and deed-of-trust.

Methodically, I went through the file on the transaction—no deed. Then, becoming concerned, I combed through the entire file drawer, thinking possibly I had misfiled it—still no deed. Then, slightly frantic, I tore through the entire file cabinet, one drawer at a time, and still failed to locate the vital paper.

A call to the escrow officer informed me it would be nearly impossible to duplicate the document as it had already been re-corded with the county. By this time I was in a nervous frenzy, desperately trying to recall the last time I had handled the deed. It had been a few days earlier, and I distinctly remembered returning the deed and file folder to the file cabinet drawer. I was unable to recall if I had returned the deed to the file folder or had possibly left it loose, on top of the folder. Because the folder is legal size, fourteen inches, and my cabinet only accommodates twelve-inch folders, I had lain it in the back part of the drawer, lengthwise, on top of several other legal-sized folders. These real estate files are all kept in the bottom drawer of the cabinet.

The only thing I could imagine was that possibly the deed had become accidentally mixed up with some newspapers and thrown out—a prospect that did nothing to calm my agitation.

After spending several frustrating hours re-searching through the file cabinet and working with my pendulum, which consistently led me back to the file cabinet, I went to bed that night exhausted.

As I was drifting off to sleep, I had an instantaneous picture flash through my mind—like a two- or three-second movie. My mind's eye saw the file drawer closed. Then, as it was being opened, the very top-most paper in the rear of the drawer was caught against the front of the cabinet and pushed off of the drawer and fell to the floor below.

Forcing myself back to a conscious state, I made myself get up out of bed, go into my office and open the bottom drawer of the file cabinet.

Placing my hand back into the space behind the drawer, I felt downwards and there, sure enough, on the carpet under the drawer was a piece of paper which was, indeed, the missing note and deed of trust.

When I called the escrow girl the next day to inform her that the emergency was over, her question was, "How in the world did you ever think to look *under* the file cabinet?" My answer to her was, "If I told you, you would never believe me!"

A few days ago, alighting from my car, I saw my neighbor, Maude, frantically tapping on her window to me. When I went to the window, she informed me, pointing to a bare finger on her left hand, that she had lost her wedding band. It was obvious that she was terribly upset over the loss.

As I had appointments that afternoon, I was unable to help, but I assured her I would come over and assist in the search the next morning.

After breakfast the following day, I went over to Maude's house. Tearfully she explained that her late husband had placed that ring on her finger fifty years ago and because of her recent weight loss the ring had become loose.

We searched through the jewel box where Maude insisted she had placed the ring a couple of weeks earlier. We searched through her clothing, closet floor, bed clothes, and every other obvious area in the bedroom where the ring might have become hidden.

Maude had become aware of the loss about a week before summoning me, and each day that the ring was gone she became more frantic, unable to eat or sleep and literally making herself sick over the incident. The day before, she informed me, she and her cleaning lady had filtered through all the dirt in her vacuum cleaner on the chance that the machine had picked up the ring.

Our search was unrewarding and, unwilling to give up, I instructed Maude to sit on her sofa, feet extended in front and head back and propped on a large pillow.

Refraining from use of the word "hypnosis," I led Maude into a light trance, instructing her to concentrate only on my voice and teaching her step-by-step relaxation. She was told to visualize the beloved ring in her mind's eye, and when she nodded yes, that she was doing this, I asked her where she saw it.

She answered thusly, "I see it in the jewel box, along with another ring I put in there." Then, after a pause she continued, "but it's not there now; it's not in the jewel box." Unable to ascertain exactly where the ring was, she concluded that it was definitely still in her home somewhere.

The following suggestion was then given to her: "Your unconscious mind knows where that ring is. You may have a dream tonight that will disclose its whereabouts. If this happens, you will force yourself to awaken and locate it. You may visualize the location of the ring as you drift off to sleep, and again, should this happen, you will immediately act upon it. Possibly, within the next few hours or days, your unconscious mind will lead you to that ring. You may find yourself doing something unusual or may find yourself in an unusual place, not altogether certain of why you are there. If and when you look upon the ring, you will *see* it, despite the fact that it may be partially hidden or obscured."

When I aroused her from the trance her phone rang, and I left.

No more than ten minutes later, I was at home washing my hands, preparing to make a sandwich, when my phone rang.

A terse, strained voice said, "Get back over here, right away!" Startled, I asked, "Who is this? Is that you, Maude?"

Rushing back over to her house, I entered to see a white, shaken Maude sitting at her dining room table. As I sat down beside her, she wordlessly picked up a large black dish sitting off to one side of the table and placed it before me. The dish was partially filled with coins, predominately nickels. There, a little to one side, nestled amongst the coins, lay Maude's white-gold, diamond wedding ring.

In shock, she described how, after getting off of the phone, she had gone to the table, sat down and picked up the black dish.

"I was looking for something in the dish," she explained. I asked her to tell me quickly, without thinking about it, what it was she was searching for in the dish, and she answered, wide-eyed, "I haven't the faintest idea!"

While soaking in the jacuzzi pool of my favorite spa one day, I became engaged in conversation with a young married couple. They were very concerned because their nine-year-old son was still wetting the bed.

"He cannot go to summer camp or have any sleepovers with his friends. The poor kid is so mortified and ashamed. We've tried everything—electronic sensors—everything. Is there any way you can help?"

Here again was untested territory, but I agreed to try. Later that afternoon they brought the boy to my home. He was a handsome youngster and very pleasant.

After explaining what I was going to do, I started the hypnotic procedure. Being extremely self-conscious, he started to giggle, but soon the giggles ended as he dropped into a trance.

I told him he would be very conscious of emptying his bladder just prior to retiring. Also, he would refrain from drinking liquids for at least an hour before going to bed. Then I stated that as the night wore on and he needed to urinate, a tiny bell would ring in his head, and he would awaken only enough to take himself to the toilet. Then, upon returning to bed, he would immediately drop back into a deep sleep. A part of his mind would always be alert, would awaken him when it was necessary.

Simple, but very effective. Ten days later his mother called me, ecstatic. He had not had an "accident" since I hypnotized him, and it looked as though he would be able to attend camp that summer.

Many times people ask, "What if you can't bring me out of the trance?" I assure them that this has never, nor would it ever, happen. However occasionally I encounter someone who is so happy and at ease in trance that they refuse to awaken on command.

This happened one time with my friend Dorothy. I had directed her to descend a flight of stairs. At the bottom was a beautiful garden in which was a pool of water. As it was warm, she went into the pool for a dip, then commenced on down the steps. Upon bringing her up out of the trance, I guided her up the stairs, around the pool, and up into consciousness. When I suggested she open her eyes, she totally ignored me. She had decided not to come out of the trance. I asked where she was and heard, "I am still in the pool!" I answered, "Fine, you can stay in the pool for exactly one minute; then you will come up out of the trance. If you do not follow these instructions, you *can never be hypnotized again!*" This threat was very effective and in less than two minutes she was wide awake.

More than we realize, we carry forth talents and skills from a previous lifetime. When researching the Millboro story, I had Charlie (Joe Nazarowski) sketch a hat that he and Becky had described to me. It was a pretty hat belonging to a matron in the town. She had worn it to church on Easter Sunday and caused quite a stir.

Charlie took the pen and pad I gave him and drew a very precise sketch of a lovely woman's hat. Thinking about this later, I wondered about Joe's ability to sketch today. So one afternoon I set a vase before him and asked him to sketch it. My seven-year-old granddaughter could have drawn a better likeness. Then I hypnotized him back into the life of Charlie and had him redraw the vase. It was a perfect sketch, down to the last detail. The realization dawned on me: Charlie was a graduate of West Point, and back in 1860, before the days of xerox machines and sophisticated cameras, it was very important that a military officer be able to sketch terrain, troops, supplies and the like. Great emphasis was placed then upon being able to sketch, and classes in the art were a very large part of the West Point curriculum. I suggested to Joe that if he had a few art lessons, most likely the talent to sketch would come to him very easily. It already resides in some part of his mind.

Likewise with foreign language. When I studied the life of Queen Christina with Marcia Simpson, I learned she understood several languages when in the role of the queen.

Christina was born in 1626, the only legitimate heir of King Gustaf Aldolph. From the time of his untimely death when she was seven, she was groomed, night and day, to become Queen of Sweden.

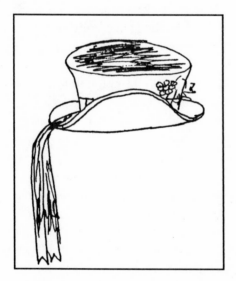

Sketch of "Ava's hat"
done by Joe when
hypnotized

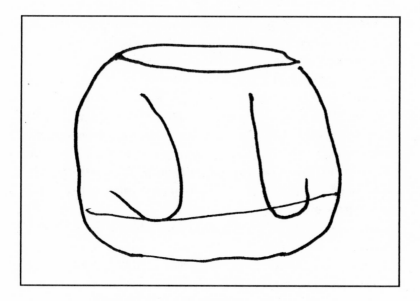

Sketch Joe made of vase when conscious

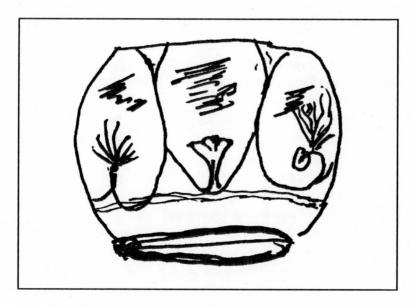

Sketch of same vase done by Joe while hypnotized

It is unknown exactly how many languages the Queen spoke— the number varies between nine and eleven. What is known is that she spoke and understood French fluently. "As a native of France," one historian reported.

Marcia today understands only English and a smattering of Spanish, as she lived for a year in South America when her father was working there. In a trance as Queen Christina, she understood Swedish, German, and especially French. When I had a friend who was born in Paris speak to her in French, the questions were carefully engineered so she could not guess at the content should she grasp a word or two.

She was instructed (in French), "Describe for us the court of Louis XIV." In English she answered, "It was dirty, smelly and very gay. The other countries were prettier but they were sterner." That is a pretty accurate appraisal of the French court at that time. Marcia said later that she was aware of much French perfume and cologne used instead of bathing. Marcia did not speak French, but the few times I tried my high-school French on her, she was quick to correct my pronunciation. Occasionally when in the role of the queen, she would speak with a definite Swedish accent.

The only persons I have worked with who spoke in a foreign language were my daughter Evie and Joann Kelley, who both regressed to Indian lifetimes in the Millboro story. Singing Bird (Evie) spoke three dialects, and Soaring Eagle (Joann) spoke only two. Sometimes Singing Bird would speak to Eagle, and he would reply, "Wrong dialect." It was amusing to watch them and hear them get to joking and bickering amongst themselves in Indian dialect. Many times they refused to translate for me, as, being lovers, their conversation took a bawdy turn.

The first time I used what I refer to as "freezing in time" was with Marcia when she, as Queen Christina, was recalcitrant about answering questions. This event is described in the following chapter.

Another time I used this ploy was when Charlie (Joe) was telling me about the holes he (and a squad of men) had drilled in the walls of the Millboro tunnel preparatory to exploding the tunnel should the Yanks invade the town. He had started to tell me the story when suddenly he stopped talking, got a strange look upon his face, and explained, "I cannot talk about this. It's military!" Knowing Charlie as I did, I realized it would be pointless to attempt to pry it out of him. I simply told him, "Freeze the entire scene in your mind. Now you are coming up through the years to the life of Joe Nazarowski. It is no longer a military secret." He spilled the entire tale, how he had been sent to Millboro, undercover, to destroy the railroad tunnel should Northern troops invade. This way they would be unable to take the engine through the tunnel to the turnaround and the Yanks would have no way to move all the supplies piled up all over the town of Millboro.

When I went with Joe and Maureen back to Millboro in 1987, I tried a ploy I call "walking hypnosis." It consists of telling the person in trance that he (or she) will open their eyes and get up and walk around. They will see everything as it is today, and also, superimposed on the scene, they will see it as it was in 1860.

This worked very well. When she was in this type of trance, I instructed Becky (Maureen) to lead us to the site of Ava's house. She took off at top speed; Joe and I could barely keep up with her. She led us down the main road, then turned off onto a small lane that had been a carriage road. One could clearly see the ruts of a small carriage. Down the small road several hundred feet, suddenly she plunged through a cluster of bushes. Hot on her trail, I plunged through the bushes after her. There, in a large clearing, was the foundation of a house.

One of the major problems when Maureen was in this state was her total lack of regard for her safety. She would plunge into the street, never looking left or right. After that, Joe and I took turns hanging onto her shirt. When conscious she explained, "I was not aware of the sound of cars; I was listening for the clop-clop of horses."

When we were searching for the area where the old stone house had stood, under which was the largest kiva in Millboro, I worked with Smokey this way. He led me through yards, across streets, right up to the lot next to the fire station. We later probed with a piece of rebar steel and hit the roof of the kiva.

Several times I had Joe lead me to various sites when he was in this type of trance. When discussing it later, he said, "It is a really weird feeling. You start to step up onto a porch step, but there's no step there!"

Some hypnotists, as well as regressing people, will sometimes take them ahead in time, perhaps to get a psychic view of the future. I hesitate to do this because, as I stated earlier in this book, a suggestion, once implanted, has a propensity to become self-actuating. And we have no way of predicting what a person will see, feel and experience when advanced in time.

Once a young man came to me with the following story. There was an entire week of his life for which he could not account. He had been heavily into drugs and suddenly experienced a lengthy blackout.

After I hypnotized him, he regressed to a period prior to the blackout. Then, one step at a time, he described to me what he was doing. He was on a bus to Laguna Beach from Anaheim. After getting off the bus, he walked around the beach for a while, made friends with some young people about his age, shared their picnic meal. Then he went home with them, in Laguna, where he stayed for three or four days. When he left, he hitchhiked to San Diego, walked around the town, saw the zoo, slept under a bridge with some homeless people. When he came out of his fugue and found himself in San Diego, he immediately hitched a ride home. Since this experience, he had been inordinately curious concerning the lost week. Later, when he was conscious, I gave him the audio tape and suggested he take it home and play it.

Several years ago, I conducted classes in "visualization for cancer." My outline was based on the book *Getting Well Again* by Doctors Carl and Stephanie Simonton. The premise behind this work is that a cancer patient (in or out of trance) could visualize the white corpuscles of the blood attacking the tumor. The goal is to persuade the body's immune system to reject the cancer. Sometimes it works miracles.

As I was preparing to conduct a class, a woman from a neighboring city called me. She had just been diagnosed with an inoperable tumor between her heart and lungs, about the size of a small grapefruit. She wanted me to work with her NOW. I suggested she wait for the class which was to start the following week. No, she wanted treatment, individually and NOW!

Relenting, I told her to come to my home the next day.

Darlene was about mid-forties, an attractive woman, exceptionally intelligent. She was an agent for the I.R.S. and did not relish her job. "It's hard," she said, "to seize people's homes and property. I was not cut out to do this." Her personal life was totally unrewarding too. She had a husband who cheated on her, and a teen-aged son who badgered her constantly for money with which to buy drugs. I explained to her that to get well, according to Simonton, she would have to turn her life around—quit her job, leave her husband, and cut off the drug-affected son. She had already left home, was living with her sister, and was on indefinite leave from the I.R.S. Her drugged-out son could not find her, and for now her life was stress-free and placid.

When she was hypnotized, I instructed her to see the white "soldiers" fighting the tumor. She said later she saw little white "pac-men" chewing on the tumor and destroying it. I continued the suggestions and closed with those geared to reinforce her self-image.

Darlene came to me for about five visits before I had to leave for Europe. Soon after I returned, she called, elated, and informed me that she was entirely cancer-free. She had undergone x-rays and a c.t. scan that had proven her to be free of malignancy.

However, there is more to this story. Before too long, Darlene's husband convinced her to move back with him, and her son was again badgering her for money. Soon, the cancer had returned, in her abdominal area. Despondent, she asked me to visit her, which I was happy to do. She was again living with her sister. Calmly she informed me that she had decided to go ahead and die. Her request to me was that I make her comfortable, control the pain, and hasten the end.

Adamantly I informed her that this is not what I do. As long as she was willing to fight, I would support her unceasingly, but if she chose to give up, she was on her own. Darlene died three months later.

One afternoon I was visiting at a friend's house. There was a young woman there, probably in her early thirties, named Sally. She mentioned that she had been adopted as a baby and was currently searching for her birth mother. She wondered if I could help her. I really did not see how I possibly could, but I agreed to try. Under hypnosis she could see her real mother very clearly. Her mother was a young girl of about eighteen. Sally said that she, as a tiny baby, was living in a hospital or some sort of home. Her birth mother came to see her on a regular basis. "When she visits, she just hold me and rocks, crying all the time." Sally felt that the girl's mother would not let her bring the baby home because she was illegitimate. "I was about six months old when my mother finally agreed to give me up. I see my mother sobbing, signing a lot of papers. Her brother is there with her; he is looking over the papers. He's a lawyer." I have no idea how Sally knew all this—perhaps babies are a lot more perceptive than we give them credit for.

Sally had been working with an organization that helps reunite birth mothers with their adopted offspring. About a week later she called to say that they had discovered her mother's name and the town in Ohio in which she had lived when Sally was born.

On a hunch of mine, we went into the local county law library and looked up the listing of lawyers in that town. Sure enough, there was a lawyer with the same name as Sally's mother. Sally placed a call to him that evening and discovered that he was, indeed, her uncle. He put her in contact with her birth mother. The

story she told under hypnosis had been generally accurate except
that the brother at the time of adoption had been a law student, not
a lawyer.

Shortly after that episode, another girl came to see me named
Gladys. She, of all things, was searching for her father. All her life
she had felt like an outsider in her family, as though she did not
belong. After she became of age, her mother finally leveled with
her, admitting she had been a married W.A.C. stationed in Hawaii
during W.W. II. She had enjoyed a brief fling with a Naval officer
she met while there which resulted in the birth of Gladys. In those
days, when a service woman became pregnant, she was immediately discharged from the service. Gladys' mother returned to the
States and gave birth. She wrote to her husband, then in the
European theater, and admitted her adultery, offering him a divorce. The husband loved his wife dearly, was willing to overlook
her escapade, and agreed to raise Gladys as his own.

Not expecting much, I hypnotized Gladys and instructed her to
see her mother while stationed in Hawaii. She was able to see her
mother, younger, in uniform. Then I suggested she see her father.
At this time I had my eyes closed and was visualizing along with
Gladys. She gasped and said, "Oh, my God, he's handsome! He
looks just like some old-time movie star I've seen." I answered,
"Tyrone Power." "Yes," she exclaimed, "that's who he looks like."

After Gladys returned to the conscious state, we discussed how
exceedingly striking the man had looked. Then she asked, "Why
doesn't he want me, why doesn't he look for me?"

My answer was, "Perhaps he doesn't even know about you.
Maybe he was sent on into combat after the affair began. Maybe he,
too, was married. Perhaps it was just not meant to be." My words
appeared to placate her

A friend of mine, Lois, had always thought she was adopted.
Because she is a dead-ringer for her father, she decided he was
either her real father or he was perhaps an uncle. Her mother had
always been something of a stranger to Lois, and the mother had

always favored the other three girls in the family, the oldest two which were hers from an earlier marriage. The third sister, Sara, was nearly Lois' age. Too close, in fact, for them both to have been born to Lois' mother.

When Lois sent back east for a copy of her birth certificate, she was not surprised to discover it had been obviously altered. Neither her mother or father would discuss it with her, nor would anyone else in either family.

One day Lois brought one of her older sisters, Ruth, to be regressed (the regression was about an entirely different matter). Ruth had no inclination of Lois' suspicions.

During the regression I asked Ruth to go back before the time of Sarah's birth. "Was her mother big, did she look pregnant?" I inquired.

"Oh, yes, she's huge. The baby will come any day now," she answered.

Then I inquired regarding Lois' birth. She looked puzzled and said, no, her mother was not big before Lois was born. In fact, someone (she did not know who) carried Lois into the house through the front door. Lois was a pretty big baby, not a newly born, when she came into the family.

Before awakening Ruth I suggested she would not remember anything that we had discussed while she was hypnotized. Ruth awakened, happy, smiling and cheerful, never knowing she had absolutely confirmed Lois' suspicions.

CHAPTER FOURTEEN

A BABY FOR QUEEN CHRISTINA

WHEN QUEEN CHRISTINA ABDICATED the throne of Sweden in 1654 to move to Rome and become a Catholic, it was generally believed that she undertook this radical change in order to avoid marriage with her cousin. Because she was given to a very masculine demeanor in both manner and dress, it was also believed that she was a lesbian. Stories of bisexuality and hermaphroditism surrounded her all her life.

Since the Queen's death in 1689, historians and biographers have speculated on the depth of her relationship with Cardinal Decio Azzolino, her long-time friend and mentor. At the end of the last century, Baron de Bildt, then the Swedish Ambassador to Rome, discovered letters written by the Queen to Azzolino which delineate clearly that for a time, at least, the Queen was deeply in love with him.

There exists today three separate categories of facts that indicate strongly that the Queen and the Cardinal became parents in the year 1666 in Hamburg, Germany. The first set of facts derive from recorded events of the time. The second group from testimony obtained through hypno-regression of a subject, Marcia Simpson Nelson, who has relived and described events of the Queen's life, and the last set of clues evolve from medical records of the Queen, which indicate a prolapsed uterus, symptomatic of a late and difficult pregnancy.

In late May of 1666, Christina left Rome for Hamburg with no fanfare. This woman, who liked to travel with an entourage of hundreds, was attended on this trip with a group of only sixteen persons. The reason for her sudden departure, suggested hesitatingly by historians, is that she was heading to Sweden in an attempt to straighten out her finances and collect monies owed her by the Swedish government.

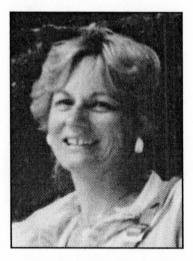

Marcia Simpson Nelson

This reasoning is offered hesitatingly because it holds no water whatsoever. For many months prior to the Queen's departing Rome, her envoy to Sweden, Count Adami, had been busy putting her affairs in order and by March, 1666, not only had her monetary accounts balanced but had succeeded in collecting a large amount of the debt owed to the Queen.

Christina and her small group literally fled to Hamburg, taking only two days longer than courier time, in itself no small feat. After arriving in Hamburg, she had several meetings with her attorney, after which she went into seclusion for several months. During these months she was reported to be almost permanently ill.

Upon studying her retinue, one finds some interesting discrepancies. It is especially noted that a doctor accompanied her to Germany in 1666. The handbook published in 1966 by the Nationalmuseum in Stockholm describes how Azzolino arranged for Christina to take his protégé, Cesare Macchiati, with her as her personal physician on her journey north. Macchiati was from the Cardinal's home town of Fermo. Except for the French physician Bourdelot, who had a great influence on Christina just prior to her abdication, the Queen had a great mistrust of doctors.

Why would she suddenly decide to take a doctor along on this expedition unless it was expected she would need one? Furthermore, any doctor that attended her would have to be one that could be trusted never to reveal this monumental secret. What better choice than a young man who was indebted to the Cardinal?

A particularly intriguing point is that Christina took with her her maid, Madam Landini, but for reasons unknown, left Captain Landini, head of her guards, behind in Rome, a circumstance most unusual. In the book, *Sybil of the North* by Faith Mackenzie (Houghton Mifflin Co., Boston and New York, 1931), the author, in describing the group that traveled north with Christina, emphasized that as Captain Landini remained in Rome, Madame Landini became involved with the Marquis Del Monte, head of Christina's household, and eventually gave birth to a baby girl as the result of the liaison. The child, Maria Landini, grew up at the Queen's court and eventually became a favored singer.

This information focuses on some interesting questions, heretofore glossed over by biographers and historians. If, in fact, Madame Landini did have an out-of-wedlock child by Del Monte while in Hamburg, what was Captain Landini's reaction to this? Bearing in mind that Landini was an Italian, an ethnic group notoriously hot-headed, did he just blithely accept the role of cuckold, give the child his name, and raise it as his own? References abound in the literature that the baby born to Landini in Hamburg that winter was fathered by Del Monte. Considering that Captain Landini calmly accepted the child, it would appear that the stories of Landini's adultery were contrived, that the Queen's child was left in Hamburg, and we know that Landini's baby went back to Rome. Hamburg was a long way from Rome and should word leak out that the group had left a child in Hamburg, it would be easy to pretend it was Landini's and that it had been necessary to surrender the child for adoption because it was illegitimate. This would camouflage the fact that it was, indeed, the Queen who had left a baby in Hamburg. Our subject in hypnosis stated that "The young girl always thought that she had been born *to a lady of the Queen."*

All three of the principles, Landini, his wife, and Del Monte, remained in the Queen's service until her death. By today's liberalized standards this would pose an impossible situation, but in the moral atmosphere of 1666, it would be utterly incredible. Indubitably, Madame Landini was pregnant prior to departing Rome and, probably given no choice, agreed to play the role of adulterous wife to camouflage the fact that the Queen was also having a baby. Indications of a carefully contrived cover-up abound, bearing the stamp of the political genius for which Azzolino was noted. Let us consider here that Azzolino was appointed Secretary of State to the Pope, second highest position in the Catholic Church, while Christina was in Hamburg having his child.

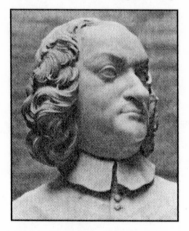

*Cardinal Decio Azzolino
by Bernini*

Let us further consider the extent of the trouble that the pair had made for themselves. A few months after her arrival in Rome, Azzolino had been forced to write a letter to the Pope assuring him that his friendship with the Queen was completely platonic. This action was necessitated by rumors and stories circulating in Rome about them, rumors that were triggered by his frequent visits to her quarters. Despite this formal protestation of innocence, the two continued to be the butt of gossip.

Had the fact of the pregnancy become public knowledge, as it most certainly would have had she remained in Rome, their world would have literally come crashing down upon them. The Pope would have had no choice but to excommunicate them both. They would have been forced to leave Rome, but where would they have gone? No Catholic country would have dared offer them sanctuary, and it is inconceivable that a Protestant country would have taken them in. If they had, by some stroke of luck, found a refuge, how would they have lived? Neither was capable of earning a living on his own—he a prince of the Church and she the Church's greatest trophy!

Christina was miserable beyond measure during those winter months in Hamburg, and this misery was aggravated by a coldness on the part of Azzolino. Sven Stolpe, in his book, *Christina of Sweden* (MacMillan Co., N.Y., 1966), describes how powerfully passionate were Christina's letters to Azzolino during this period, and he further relates that Azzolino's attitude was that of a person attempting to cool a relationship. Stolpe believes that the two had had a happy, stormless friendship, prior to the Hamburg expedition, which had for some "unknown" reason ended. The reason, of course, being the baby. He discouraged her return to Rome, even worked in vain to secure for her the throne of Poland which had been recently vacated. Gribble, in *The Court of Queen Christina of Sweden* (London), suggests that Azzolino's sensual passion for the Queen had, at some stage in their relationship, been transformed into a purely spiritual passion, and this before she had wished it. Later he elaborates that there had been trouble—a quarrel or estrangement—after which his passion cooled and she continued to love for a time until eventually her passion evolved into deep friendship.

In the following spring, Machiatti wrote to the Cardinal that Christina's problems had transposed themselves from the physical to the emotional, and he was convinced her poor frame of mind was responsible for her continued illnesses.

Christina threatened suicide, wrote to the Cardinal that as she had lost everything that made life pleasant, she no longer wished to live and in every way displayed all the symptoms of a severe post-partum depression.

Portraits of the Queen display a radical body change between the ages of thirty-five and forty-one. A painting done of Christina when she was thirty-five portrays a slender, svelte, vivacious,

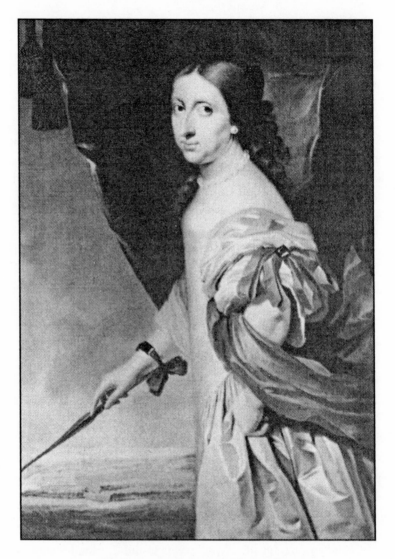

Christina at the age of thirty-five,
painted by A. Wauchters in Norrköping in 1661,
where the Queen stayed shortly after the death of Charles X.
A thin, sprightly Queen,
painted a few years prior to her pregnancy.

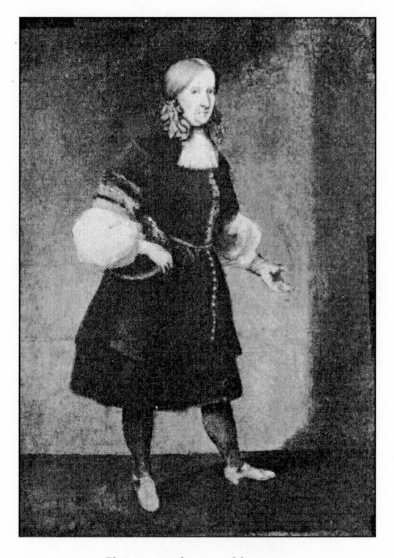

Christina at the age of forty-one,
attributed to W. Heimbach.
A dumpy, matronly looking Queen
painted shortly after the birth of her child.

sharp-eyed woman possessed of a quick restlessness. Studying a portrait done at age forty-one, it is difficult to conceive it is the same person. We see a dumpy, matronly, placid little woman. Many women undergo a radical body change in a few years, and this change is frequently precipitated and expedited by childbirth.

About half way through our hypno-regressive experiments, the idea that the Queen had gone to Hamburg to give birth began to evolve. The more one studies her life, the more obvious it becomes that the ill-fated trip in 1666 was due to an unexpected pregnancy.

At one juncture, we placed our subject into the Queen's life at age sixty-two and inquired at what age the Queen had been when she had had the baby. The response was even more surprising than anticipated. Her extreme distress and agitation assured us we had hit a nerve. We then placed her at age forty, telling her she was in Hamburg, it was early December, and she had been ill. Her teeth chattering so badly she could scarcely speak, she described the freezing cold the Queen was experiencing. Later she told of extreme pressure and that the pain went on for many hours and she did not know night from day.

All efforts to get her to admit to having a baby drew a blank. We instructed her to freeze the entire picture in her mind, then we brought her forward through the years to her present lifetime, "where there is no threat!" This technique worked, and she described the birth of the child for us in detail.

She said the room was warmer now, everyone with the Queen was very worried, and that the room smelled rank. The Queen, she continued, was yelling and cursing her maids because they were holding her down and pushing her legs up. (Christina was known for swearing like a dockhand when motivated.) She said there was straw all over the floor of the room, put there as insulation. Medical doctors agree that straw was used in delivery rooms in the seventeenth century and earlier, both as insulation and as a measure of cleanliness. An exhaustive search of the literature revealed that in the late 1500s, straw covered the floor of the Hotel Dieu in Paris, a

1200-bed hospital *(Eternal Eve* by Harvey Grahan, Doubleday, 1951).

Our subject added that the Queen never consciously accepted the fact that she had a child, that her attendants whisked the child out of the room immediately and that it was never seen or acknowledged by Christina. Her biographers tell us that Christina was a master at interpreting facts her own way, that she saw only what she chose to see and believed what she preferred to believe. Later our subject said that the child had been a girl and had been adopted by an upper-middle-class family in Hamburg. She added that the girl always had her own money, as the Queen's advisors (Azzolino) arranged, through attorneys, for money to be sent to the girl.

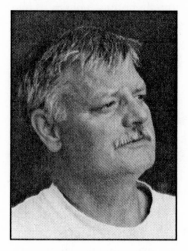

The late Kent Montin, Ph.D., who contributed much to this research, courtesy of Leif Montin

Dr. Kent Montin, of the Psychology Department of Uppsula University in Sweden, witnessed a hypnotic session with our subject. At his suggestion, we conducted a "psycho-drama" which consisted of him taking the role of Azzolino and talking to the hypnotized Queen while in that role. They discussed the impending baby, and he reminded her that the birth must be kept secret. This statement evoked a good deal of emotion in the "queen." Shaking her finger at him, she stated firmly, "You cannot make me feel guilty. You are a man of God and you had a large part in it!" Then she expressed her fear, claiming, "There's too many people who have to be trusted." When Dr. Montin mentioned something regarding the family who would raise the child, she cut him off tersely with, "I do not want to know!" When the matter of money was raised she said, "It must come from my funds; I want it through my funds."

Later in that session, Montin asked our "queen" if there had been more than one child. This she denied. He then reported to the group watching the experiment that upon hearing about our findings regarding the baby, a group of historians from Uppsula University, north of Stockholm, had searched through the Queen's financial records in the Vatican and determined that Christina did, in fact, send money on a regular basis, until her death, to a girl in Hamburg. This convinced them that there had, most certainly, been a child.

Other findings unearthed during the study of her financial records gave them reason to suspect that there may have been two or possibly three children born to Christina during her lifetime. This theory is easily discounted by the fact that never, at any time in her mature life, was Christina out of the public eye long enough to have borne a child, except for the two fateful years in Hamburg in 1666.

Perhaps the most damning piece of evidence regarding Christina's pregnancy is the fact of her prolapsed uterus. Stolpe, in his book, *Fran Stocicism Till Mystick, Studier I Drotting Kristinas Maximer* (1959), describes how Christina, at the advent of the prolapse, thought she was undergoing a sex change and confided this fact to several persons. However, as the condition worsened, her doctor diagnosed a prolapse of the uterus. It is described in Stolpe's book how the uterus protruded from the vaginal opening like a pipe, resembling a penis, and this is what caused her to think she was developing masculine genital characteristics.

Dr. Ed Stone, Ob., Gyn., Orange, California, when recently interviewed said the accepted cause in the majority of cases of prolapsed uterus is obstetrical trauma. Other possible causes could be a tumor pressing against the uterus or a severe blow or fall. Heritage can predispose a woman to a prolapsed uterus, particularly if she has borne several children. Stolpe believes that Christina was a virgin all her life, and that prolapsed uterus in a virgin differs from that of a woman who has given birth. While not ruling out this possibility, Dr. Stone stated that in all his many years of practice, he has never observed a prolapse in a virgin, and he considers that this happens very rarely, if at all.

Reinforcing these views is Dr. Charles Helsel, Ob., Gyn., Lake Elsinore, California. In a written interview, Dr. Helsel said that he has observed uterine prolapse very rarely in women who have not borne children and never in a virgin. He elaborated that while it is possible to have a prolapse without having had a pregnancy, still, the common cause of prolapse is a difficult delivery. He feels that there is at least an eighty percent chance that Christina did, at some time in her life, have a child.

Medical records of the Queen make no mention of an abdominal tumor, and there is no report of her suffering an accident or fall severe enough to precipitate a uterine prolapse.

When we asked our hypnotized subject about the prolapsed uterus in her fifty-fifth year, she said that she felt tired, that her legs still bothered her, and that she had trouble walking at times. She elaborated, "I bind my stomach and it holds everything high so I don't have the pain." We inquired if the pain was caused by a prolapsed uterus and she reiterated, "It holds *everything* up." She explained that her stomach was wrapped with a piece of cloth and her maids pinned it tightly, thus resembling a girdle. Later she stated that the Queen had very bad legs, that the uterus gave her a lot of trouble, and it hurt the Queen to walk. "She is very slow and heavy."

There are many references in the literature to the Queen's weight in her later years, to her slow, waddling gait and to the fact that she always wore a wide belt or sash drawn very tightly over the lower part of the stomach, emphasizing its roundness. Both Stolpe and Georgina Masson *(Queen Christina,* Farar, Straus & Giroux, NY, 1969), among others, make specific mention of her wearing of a wide band to support her stomach.

Medical books contain remarks on the use, in the sixteenth and seventeenth centuries, of "utero-abdominal supporters" as treatment for a prolapsed uterus. In *Eternal Eve* and again in *Iconographia Gyniatrica* (Philadelphia, 1873), utero-abdominal supporters are mentioned along with pessaries, tampons, douches and various other applications as being used as a means of offering relief.

Of course, there is no written record of a child being delivered by Queen Christina in Hamburg in 1666. This was a situation that had to be covered up at all or any costs, as exposure would have absolutely destroyed the principals and perhaps their followers. There exists, however, a plethora of clues that indicate that such a birth did occur. Lack of records documenting the birth does not, in any way, prove that it did not actually happen.

CHAPTER FIFTEEN

STROKE STRATEGY

THIS CHAPTER IS DEDICATED to the memory of the late Ray Conniff, whose beautiful music will be with us forever.

Around 1773 Anton Mesmer, in Paris, was fascinating Europe with his use of magnets to effect cures. As people taking his "cure" invariably entered a trance state, the name Mesmer became associated with hypnotism. Hence the term "mesmerism." Because of Mesmer's showmanship tactics his retreat soon became an extravaganza with a circus-like atmosphere. Sensationalism soon overcame any legitimate cures he was effecting, and his practice was decried as quackery. This was the end of Mesmer's career.

At the time of Mesmer, a priest, Father Gassner, was causing a commotion in Germany with spectacular cures. Equally as dramatic as Mesmer, Gassner seated his patients in a darkened room lighted with only a candle. After a few minutes the priest would enter the room with outstretched arms, bearing a bejeweled crucifix. In a thunderous voice he would intone a hypnotic induction resulting in the patient dropping into a deep trance. Then he would order the "evil spirits" from the victim's body.

In his most colorful experiment he placed a young girl into deep trance and informed her that her pulse would become very slow. Then he directed that her pulse would beat even more slowly and finally cease and that she would die temporarily. A nervous physician was witnessing this event. Very concerned, he took her

155

pulse and announced her *dead!* Gassner immediately commenced
to say the words, in a low and steady voice, that would restore her
to consciousness. She sat up, displaying no ill effect from her
adventure. It is said that Father Gassner never again attempted this
feat!

The man whose work best exemplifies the interworking between the mind and body was a Scottish physician named James
Esdaile. Esdaile was a surgeon in the British Army in the mid-
1800s when he was sent to India. Upon arrival he was stationed in
an outlying medical clinic near a village called "Hooghly," treating
the natives. Because he was unfamiliar with the Indian dialect, he
had a great many assistants who would translate what he said. As he
did not speak the language and was unable to talk the patients into
a trance, he soon discovered that hand passes over the body would
eventually result in the desired trance state. His assistants learned
to pass their hands over the patients, starting at their heads and
proceeding over the body to the stomach. Sometimes it would take
his workers several hours to get patients into the proper state of
trance, that state being a type of coma that is today referred to as an
"Esdaile trance."

Esdaile, in his book, *Mesmerism in India,* describes the process: "They (his workers) desire him to lie down, shut his eyes and
try to sleep, and they pass their hands slowly over the most
sensitive parts of the body." In another chapter he describes the
awakening process: "Awoke him in a few minutes, by rapid trans-
verse passes, blowing in his face and giving water to drink."

While using hand passes, the hands were held in a claw-like
position and sort of combed the area of the face and stomach, up
and down in a combing gesture. Esdaile was not aware of the field
of electricity that surrounds all living things. In my opinion it is
stroking, or combing, of that aura that induces trance.

When his workers had the patient at the desired level of trance,
the doctor would perform amputations, abdominal surgery, and
suturing. It has been reported that he performed over three hundred

MESMERISM
IN INDIA

AND ITS

PRACTICAL APPLICATION IN SURGERY
AND MEDICINE

JAMES ESDAILE

"I rather choose to endure the wounds of those darts which envy cas-
teth at novelty, than to go on safely and sleepily in the easy ways of ancient mistakings – RALEIGH.

ASIAN EDUCATIONAL SERVICES
NEW DELHI ★ MADRAS ★ 1989

Title page of Dr. Esdaile's book in reprint

abdominal surgeries and several hundred minor surgeries while patients were in this state of trance. Some of the tumors Esdaile removed weighed as much as 80 pounds. His mortality rate was an unheard of five percent at a time when fifty percent was the norm. Bear in mind this occurred prior to 1850, when even ether had not been recognized as an anesthetic.

Throughout my work with stroke patients I marvelled that the majority lent themselves so well and so quickly to the trance state. Esdaile explains this several times in his book: "I am now able to say from experience that debility of the nervous system predisposes to the easy reception of the mesmeric (the term hypnotism was yet to be coined) influence, and I augur well of a patient's power of submission, when I recognize in him the listless air, 'l'air abattu,' that usually accompanies functional debility of the nerves." Esdaile considered mesmerism, in itself, in some cases to be a medical agent. He states, "I was certain . . . that in the mesmeric trance, the muscles of the whole body had been as plastic, and obedient to my command, as clay in the hands of the potter; and I felt satisfied that if the same state of things could be brought about, muscular spasms and contractions would disappear before this great solvent. The straightening of limbs, long contracted, very soon verified this influence."

The doctor closed his book with the following statements regarding mesmerism:

> From the foregoing facts it is allowable to conclude, I hope, that Mesmerism is a natural power of the human body. That it effects directly the nervous and muscular systems. That in the mesmeric trance the most severe and protracted operations can be performed, without the patients being sensible of the pain.
>
> That spasms and nervous pain often disappear before the mesmeric trance.
>
> That it gives us a complete command of the muscular system, and is therefore of great service in restoring contracted limbs.
>
> That the chronic administration of mesmerism often acts as a useful stimulant in functional debility of the nerves.

> That as sleep, in the absence of pain, is the best condition of the system for subduing inflammation, the mesmeric trance will probably be found to be a powerful remedy in local inflammations.
>
> That the imagination has nothing to do with the first physical impression made on the system by mesmerism, as practiced by me.
>
> That it is not necessary for the eyes to be open: I always shut them as a source of distraction; and blind men are as readily mesmerised as others. . . .

Esdaile echoed one of my favorite statements as regards skeptics of hypnotism, "There is none so blind as he who WILL not see!"

Esdaile had the idea that the trance was inspired by an exchange of some sort of body fluids between the hypnotist and the subject. He refers to getting the practitioner's sweat on the subject and blowing on his eyes and face. More recent opinion is that the mesmerizer is "stroking" the subject's aura. I found the "sweat" idea disgusting and that blowing on the subject's face and eyes only irritated them.

THE NERVOUS SYSTEM

The nervous system is divided into two main parts: the Central Nervous System (CNS) and the Autonomic Nervous System (ANS). The CNS controls organs under voluntary control while the ANS regulates individual organ function and homeostasis.

Heart rate, dilation of blood vessels, visual accommodation, bowels, bladder control are but a few tasks monitored by the ANS. For the most part the ANS is not subject to voluntary control. However, it has been proven time and time again that persons in a trance state can, either by themselves or led by a hypnotist, influence the behavior of the ANS.

The nature of the human body is to attempt to heal itself. It has been established that when brain cells become damaged, adjoining cells eventually take over the duties of the damaged cells. Slowly, over the years, the thought came into my head that we might be able to manipulate the ANS to restore some movement and limited use of limbs to a paralyzed stroke patient.

Visiting a local "Stroke Club" I recruited a couple of volunteers. I explained very carefully to them that this research was extremely experimental and the only thing I could guarantee them was that it would cause no harm or further damage. They did not care if it was experimental! They had been assured by doctors that they would probably never get any better and could look forward to a lifetime of semi-invalidism.

Because most stroke patients invariably suffer brain damage to some degree, I figured it would take several sessions to get them into any state of trance.

Not so! At least with the first person I worked with. So far it has been utterly amazing how readily this person responded to the hypnotic induction and suggestion. To date I have taken most of my clues from my clients.

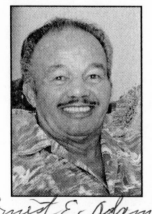

ERNIE ADAMS

My first stroke victim was Ernie Adams. When Ernie hobbled over to where I was sitting after having asked for volunteers, my heart sank. His left hand was frozen in a claw shape, his left arm was bent with his hand near his face. He walked with great difficulty and all movement was stiff. Thinking, "There's no way on earth I am ever going to be able to help this man," I took his name and phone number and promised to call him.

Ernie is sixty-eight years old and was a landscape designer before he became ill. About three years prior to our meeting, he had been in a serious car accident and sustained an injury to his neck.

While he was undergoing surgery on his neck, the stroke hit. It traveled sidewise across his chest and up and down his entire backbone, damaging all the nerves in its wake. Doctors worked almost two hours to save his life. When he finally awakened, he was in a fetal position, his left hand frozen like a claw, arm bent, hand near his face. It took four men to lift him into his bed. As soon as possible he began intensive therapy which he underwent for two years. At the end of this time he was informed that further therapy was pointless.

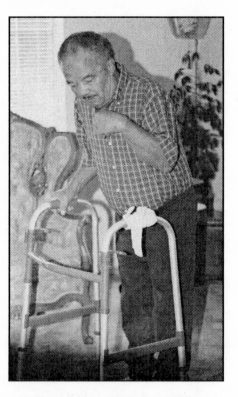

Ernie as he looked prior to the hypnotherapy.

Shortly after I began his first session, he dropped into a deep trance. I proceeded to give him healing suggestions, i.e., a warm, healing light is encircling his entire body, traveling up and down his back, encircling and energizing his CNS. Then the light massaged his left shoulder, traveled slowly down his arm, and worked on each individual finger. When Ernie awoke from the trance he gave me a large grin and announced, "When the light went down my arm, I could feel my arm twitching." This thrilled and excited me because I realized that we were getting some response, however slight. Later Ernie announced that almost immediately after the first session he discovered he could move the fingers on his left hand. Then he added, "I wish someone would take the muscles in my shoulder and arm and just pull them!"

In our next session this is exactly what we did. I suggested to him that the healing light divided into two parts, and one pulled on one end of the muscle and the other on the other end. Then we pulled the nerves, strengthening and revitalizing them.

At the beginning of the next session I told him to see and feel the light moving back and forth over his left shoulder, over all his muscles. Nerves, bones, sinews, cells in the shoulder responding to the light, informing him that he may feel a tingling or twitching in the shoulder and arm.

It was suggested that he picture himself as well, as he was prior to the stroke. While he was hypnotized, I asked him to bend his elbow, which he did. Then I had him work it back and forth, feeling it become more and more limber as the muscles and nerves loosened up.

In the third session we had the light travel over his body, then concentrate on blood flowing freely through the shoulder and arm. Then we worked on the brain cells, instructing healthy cells to assume the duties of the damaged cells.

Sometime around his third or fourth session, he amazed me by flexing and rotating his left shoulder. Then, when hypnotized, I told him to relax his left hand, open his fingers, raise his arm, and then bring it down slowly. Putting a tennis ball directly under his descending hand, I told him to close his fingers around the ball— he did. After squeezing the ball, he lifted it, and I suggested he throw it. He tried; it sort of dribbled down his arm. Later I had him flatten out his hand on a clip board and raise one finger at a time. He did amazingly well for a man whose hand, a few weeks earlier, had been frozen into the shape of a claw.

The next session Ernie raised his T-shirt and flexed the muscles of his stomach, grinning his disarming smile. I had not even been aware that his stomach muscles were frozen solid.

During his sixth session I directed the blood to flow heavily and freely into his left arm and leg. They were swollen. We worked on the circulation and by the session's end, they were normal. He said his bowels and bladder were now straightened out. He "gets a feeling" when it's time to urinate and move bowels.

Then he really shocked me by saying that his arms and hands were sore because the previous day he had worked in the yard, pruning trees and bushes.

Ernie no longer walks with a cane. He sleeps a lot better and says the hypnosis helped his mind adjust to the damage done to his body. The feeling is rapidly returning to his left leg and hand. Now he is even able to pick up and take his pills, something he would not have been able to attempt before. Laughingly, he stated, "They scatter all over the table, and I drop about half of them, but eventually I take five dirty pills." It was easier each time he did it, he added.

Just a little thing like being able to wear a wrist watch was a thrill for him. Until then his arm and wrist had been too swollen to tolerate a watch.

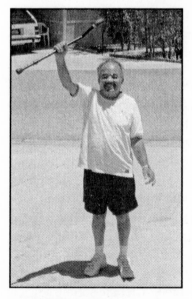

A jubilant Ernie waves the cane (which he no longer needs) over his head.

Again I asked him to squeeze the tennis ball—this was about our seventh meeting. As he was squeezing the ball, I suggested he raise and lower his hand, bending the arm at the elbow. Next I asked him to throw the ball. He did. It flew across the office, hitting a metal dish on my desk and knocking it off. The racket that ensued scared both of us and almost brought him out of the trance. No damage was done, and if I try that again in the future I will first move anything that might be in the way.

What Delene, Ernie's wife, noticed almost immediately after

the first hypnosis session was the change in Ernie's disposition and personality. He immediately became cheerful, optimistic, and pleasant to be around. Before he had snapped at her constantly. As she stated, "Anything I said, he literally snapped my head off!"

Right about this time I decided there was not much more I could do for Ernie. He had become used to the weekly sessions, really built up a dependence upon them. I told him he had graduated. Seeing the disappointment on his face, it was suggested that he get a small notebook, keep a record of any new problems that occurred, and in about three weeks he could come for a "post-graduate" booster session. He grabbed onto that idea, and within a few months I expect Ernie to be weaned off the hypnosis and handling any ensuing problems alone.

BOB JENKINS

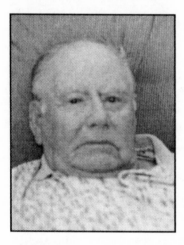

After signing up Ernie to partake in my experiment I talked to Bob Jenkins. Bob is an eighty-two-year-old man who sits on the board of directors of several banks, some of which he started. His stroke occurred in December of 2001 and was, when we started, about six months old. His whole left side was paralyzed and after several months of therapy, he was told his prognosis for getting better was very poor.

Bob, like Ernie, responded very well. After the first session, he could move his fingers for the first time. After the second session he had conflicting appointments, and I did not see him for a few weeks.

I was invited to speak before the local Stroke Support Group, and imagine my shock and surprise when I spotted Bob at the back of the room reaching across the table with his *left* arm to pick up something. This is when it dawned on me that the hypnotic suggestions keep on working even when they are not consistently reinforced.

At that meeting he described to me how he had been asleep a couple of nights previously. His feet had become very cold so he imagined the warm white light going to his feet, and it warmed them up.

At an earlier session Bob had interrupted me with "The light is too hot; it's burning me." Surprised, I told him I would turn down the heat in the light. Then I said we would put a gauge in the light so he could adjust the temperature any way he liked. Bob placed a lot of stock in that light.

There were three more sessions with Bob during which he made amazing progress. After about the fourth meeting, he showed me the papers he had obtained from the Department of Motor Vehicles and announced that he was going to get his driver's license back that week. He was still dependent upon a cane and not using his left hand and arm with much dexterity. I urged him to wait for a few weeks. Of course he did not, and he greeted me at our next meeting with a few well chosen words for the Motor Vehicle Department.

Bob Jenkins seems to regard his life-threatening stroke as a major inconvenience in his life. At the rate he is recovering I am not so sure that his is a bad mind-set.

The last time I saw Bob he was walking around the room in a steady, confident way. I gave him the same advice I had given Ernie. "When you go out, take your cane and put it in the back of the car so you will always have it handy. Whenever you can walk without it, do so. If the terrain is rough, use it. Soon you will no longer depend upon it. I saw Bob recently and he appeared to be entirely functional.

WALTER HOPP

Walter is a seventy-seven-year-old man who had a stroke three years ago. He suffered no paralysis (that I know about) and appears to be in excellent health physically. However, Walter suffers from aphasia, which means he cannot speak.

I worked with Walter for five sessions, tried everything I could think of to restore his voice, to no avail. The usual suggestions that seem to work so well with paralyzed persons failed to help Walter at all. After the fifth session, we discussed this and agreed that further sessions were pointless. Recently I heard that the doctors have reexamined Walter and discovered that he does not have aphasia. It is my understanding that they are trying a new type of treatment, possibly surgery.

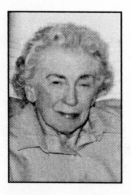

JUNE BACA

June is a seventy-eight-year-old woman who suffered the first of four strokes in 1956 at the age of thirty-five. She had successive attacks in 1961, 1995, and 1996. Her entire body was pretty well ravaged by the strokes. After the third stroke she suffered severely from migraine headaches, and after the 1996 attack the migraines disappeared.

After giving her extensive suggestions for five sessions and seeing no improvement, I told her that in my opinion the hypnosis was not helping and that we should probably terminate the treatment. It upset me to tell her this because June is an adorable woman—petite, cheerful, upbeat, with a delightful personality.

As I expected, she became extremely upset when I tried to stop the work, exclaiming, "But my right leg is still paralyzed." Relenting, I agreed to see her the following week.

Wednesday came and my doorbell rang. There was Ben, June's husband, standing at the door. When I asked where June was, he pointed to the car and announced, "She's coming."

I looked down the driveway and there was June, climbing out of the car unassisted. Then she walked slowly, but very steadily, toward the house, using no cane.

I could not believe my eyes. She climbed the stairs of the porch, entered the house, to all appearances very normal. We talked a while, and I asked them to return the next week, which they happily did.

I took videotape of June walking up the driveway, ascending the stairs, entering the house. Further tape was taken of her moving fingers on both hands, moving arms, both legs, and bending in the middle. Grinning widely, her only complaint was that her right leg was still a little stiff.

Ben announced that she had insisted upon a long walk a few nights previously, and then the next day, at her insistence, he had taken her to the local mall. There, while he sat and read the paper, she walked up and down the mall several times. I told June that she had just graduated with highest honors. Go figure!

RAY CONNIFF

Ray Conniff was in Palm Springs, California, attending a jazz festival and to receive an award when he was hit with a massive stroke. The date was March 22, 2002.

After his release from the hospital, Ray and Vera, his wife, took up residence in Palm Springs so he could have access to the Palm Springs Stroke Center—a unique, one-of-a-kind institution built and supported by both volunteer funds and workers. The center has every facility imaginable to help victims of strokes. A fairly spacious building, there are two rooms of exercise equipment, a large auditorium (donated by Paul and Joann Newman),

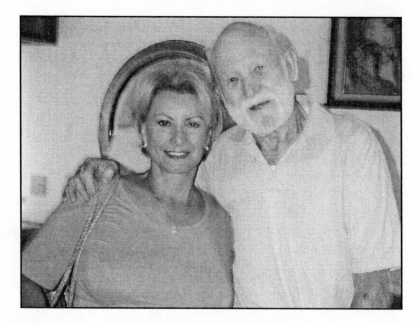

Ray Conniff and his wife Vera

game rooms, a thrift shop, a very large dining room, and other features too numerous to mention.

Ray and Vera spent every day at the Stroke Center where they heard about the hypnosis experiment I was conducting. Vera wanted to try it immediately but Ray held off for several weeks as his religion advocated strongly against hypnosis. Finally Vera persuaded Ray to try it, and she called for an appointment. Fortunately I had just finished with Walter Hopp so I was able to work with Ray.

When he came to the house, I was shocked. Ray towered over all of us, easily six-foot, four or five inches tall. And also Ray was very, very thin. Mostly I was impressed by how terribly weak he appeared. Vera practically lifted him out of the car and carried him into the house. He tried to walk, but his left foot just dragged along the driveway.

Ray fought the hypnosis the first couple of sessions, but, even though he had reservations, the first session was successful in that his bladder immediately came under control. By the third meeting Ray had decided he was not going against God and became very involved. Vera said he looked forward all week to our sessions. After the fourth week, Ray was like a new man—much stronger, eyes bright, gregarious and out-going. Vera was thrilled when his bladder came under control, but she was even more excited when, after four meetings, he was strong enough to pull himself up, walk to the bathroom by himself, and attend to his needs. Before long he was able to raise his left leg and walk fairly normally with a cane.

During our final meeting Ray proudly showed me how he could move his left thumb and forefinger. It is my belief that if Ray had survived, he would have become, within a few weeks, fully functional. I last saw Ray on Wednesday, October 9th. On Saturday, October 12th, Ray passed away in the San Diego area.

DIANE BINGHAM

Diane is a fifty-four-year-old woman who, prior to her stroke, was a food service manager for the local school district. Her stroke left her right side paralyzed. When she came to me, her right arm was in a brace, her hand, frozen into a "fist," was in a separate brace.

She was given the usual suggestions—that the healing light traveled over her shoulder, arm, and hand. Her right leg seemed to be in good shape; she had no trouble walking unaided by a cane or walker. However, she did what a lot of stroke victims do—instead of planting her foot on the ground heel first, which is the normal way to walk, she drops her toes first, making her gait clumsy.

When she started, she had no peripheral feeling in her shoulder, arm, or hand. After the first session, she arrived with the brace off of her arm and told me she had feeling in her arm. No control,

Dana Bingham

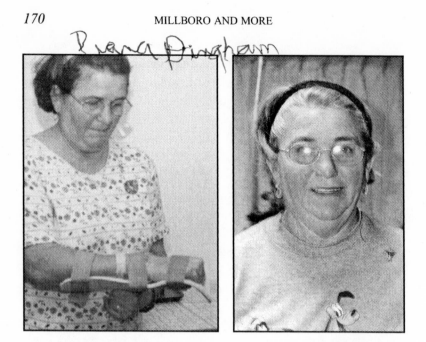

Diane's arm and hand in brace   *Diane Bingham*

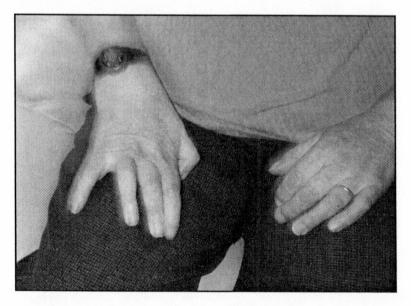

Diane's right hand, locked in a fist for five years, unfolds

just feeling, which I verified with a pin prick. The next week the feeling had spread into her hand, which is no longer frozen into a fist. It is partially extended. It has been five years since Diane's stroke. Restoring the feeling into her arm, hand, and shoulder is a good start. She has received suggestions regarding an increase in circulation and this has proved to be effective. At this writing, her outlook is good, as is her morale.

MADELINA DE PAZ

My introduction to Madelina de Paz was through my publisher, Paul Clemens. When he discovered I was writing a chapter relating to stroke victims, he suggested I contact her. Madelina had written a book called *Stroke: Brain-Assault,* which Paul published in 2002.

As she had recently moved to the Los Angeles area, I had no trouble locating her by phone. A couple of week later, Madelina's son drove her out to meet me. When she got out of the car to come into the house, my heart went out to her. Madelina is a tiny little thing, and it was heart wrenching to watch her try to walk, dragging along one leg, encased in a brace.

Madelina was born in the Philippine Islands and, after completing her education, moved to the United States. Her primary occupation is that of nuclear engineer in which she was engaged when her stroke hit twelve years ago. The stroke devastated her body, and she spent many years in therapy and rehabilitation.

Over the years she devised a series of exercises which helped, somewhat, in her recovery to this point. In her book she describes in exquisite detail each exercise and how it should be done. She also explains the working of the brain and what happens when a stroke occurs.

Madelina took to hypnosis like a duck takes to water. Her right leg, ankle and foot and right arm and hand were ice cold and hard as a rock. It was as if they had been in a freezer for a month. I started with the pin-prick routine, although I knew there was no feeling in either limb. Then I suggested that the blood flow freely into her arm and leg, rapidly, congregating there and warming the limbs and "thawing them out!"

After the second session, her affected limbs were soft and warm to the touch. The peripheral feeling had returned. After a few more sessions, Madelina developed feeling in her leg and could bend her knee. Also there was feeling and sensation in her arm—no control, just a strong reaction. Every time I hypnotized her, her right arm would involuntarily raise up high, away from her body, and wave in the air.

At a later time she awoke to find her right leg moving. As she watched, her right foot was moving from left to right using the heel

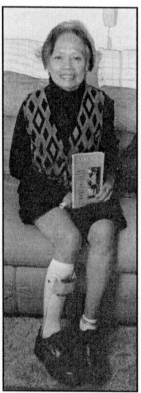

Madelina when I first met her— she is holding her book.

Madelina recently demonstrated her "miracle" for me—she walked with no support.

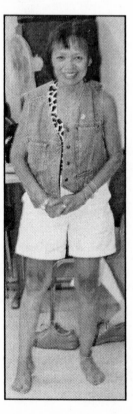

as a base point. She reports that the blood circulation in the right side of her body has been excellent since the hypnosis. She can bend her right wrist with the help of her left hand, a feat that was impossible before.

Following is a letter Madelina sent me:

"I took off my shoes, ankle and leg brace. I massaged my right toes and foot. I checked my right foot and found it was flat on the floor. I hung onto my walker and concentrated on taking the first step. I felt so good I took the next step, and the next, and the next. I walked with the walker, with no brace or other support, for one hundred eighty-four feet. It is a feat!

"Less than two weeks later a miracle happened. I tried to see if I could walk with no support—no brace, no walker. Surprise of my life—I can walk! What I did was concentrate. For every step, I check that my foot is flat and my ankle is straight; then I act. It's slow walking but a huge accomplishment after twelve years of being unable to walk.

"The physical improvement is incredible. I attribute my achievement to hypnosis which I did not know anything about, until that day in February when you introduced hypnosis to me. Hypnosis makes me realize that our mind is alert. And it gives us an option to achieve what we cannot achieve via common ways. Hypnosis focuses on outside of ourselves, changes behavior, and we enter an altered state and receive suggestions. When experiencing hypnosis, the hypnotic subject is in control. The hypnotherapist makes suggestions. Most people are skeptical of hypnosis because the unknown and uncertainties are nerve-wracking. A friend of mine was not comfortable with hypnosis, until yesterday when we talked about it for an hour. To ease up any doubts and answer her questions, I advised her to read and learn about it. How great it is— to know the amazing, beautiful mind!"

Madelina is a study in tenacity. I predict, with her determination, she will be fully functional before too many more months. One of her immediate goals is to write another book documenting her "amazing recover through hypnosis!"

Several people have asked why no one has used hypnosis with stroke victims before. Perhaps someone has. If so, it has been a well-guarded secret. My guess is that it has never been considered to be an effective treatment. However, recently I discovered the following website: http://my.webmo.com/content/article/45/30. It contains a lengthy article concerning stroke treatments and mentions hypnotherapy as a relaxation technique. It also states that acupuncture is endorsed by the World Health Organization as a viable stroke rehabilitation therapy.

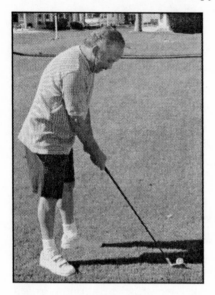

Ernie displays his golfing skills

Ernie Adams is definitely the "poster boy" for this research. In a few short weeks he went from a totally crippled, disabled, helpless victim to a fully functional human being. About eight weeks after he was released from this study, I visited him in his home. He took me outside so I could watch him prune trees and bushes. Then he took several graceful, coordinated swings with a golf club. His wife Delene gave me a list of improvements she had noticed in him. His bowel and bladder function are normal, he walks without a cane and has good balance, circulation of his blood is almost normal, and he exudes self-confidence, and his hand mobility is nearly as it was prior to the stroke. She added that she was very surprised when he volunteered to lead the exercise class at the local stroke club for a while.

Generally I do not use the word "recovered" when discussing improved stroke victims. Most patients never fully recover from a serious stroke. The word "functional" is more appropriate.

Of nine patients I worked with, all but four showed discernible improvement. One of the four was Walter Hopp whose stroke left him with an undiagnosed throat condition. The other three subjects, although unresponsive to the suggestions regarding their arms and hands, all admitted that they were fully able, after the hypnosis, to raise and lower the affected leg. Needless to say, this improved their ability to walk and climb stairs considerably.

It has been my experience that the paralyzed arm of a stroke victim has a tendency to drop out of the shoulder socket if it is not supported. This can be rectified in a couple of ways. The arm bone can be replaced into the socket by a doctor, who will then tape it into place. Or the arm can be supported by a sling or a brace. Support of some type should be given the arm as soon as possible when working with a paralyzed person.

It is possible that this type of therapy could be effectively done with groups. In my practice I have successfully entranced groups many times. Also, it is possible that this type of therapy might benefit paraplegics, quadriplegics and others paralyzed by accidents.

While the hypnosis treatment does not work with everyone, it does help enough people to definitely be considered as a viable therapy tool. Despite the fact that this study was conducted over only a few months and with only nine participants, some of the results have been so astonishing that, in my opinion, hypnosis should never be ruled out as a possible treatment for stroke paralysis.

SECONDARY GAIN

My first experience with "secondary gain" in action was several years ago when I lived in a town that was built on a sulphur water springs and was, at one time, a very popular spa center. Many famous and wealthy people used to visit the place on a regular basis to "take the waters."

One of the more popular spas was near my home, and I spent a lot of time there. I made friends with an attractive woman, fiftyish, who had suffered a stroke. She walked with a cane and could not use her left hand or arm when I first met her. She exercised in the pool every day. After several months, maybe a year, I and several others noticed that Barbara was almost normal. It appeared that she had full use of her left arm and hand, she no longer used a cane, and the slight limp in her walk was barely noticeable. Of course, we mentioned it to her. As a matter of fact, we raved about her apparent recovery. A few days later, Barbara appeared at the spa, limping severely, using a cane, and favoring her left arm and hand.

After questioning a few people who knew her better than I did, I discovered that many people in town had been doing a lot for Barbara. The Federal Government was subsidizing building a home for her. Some folks taxied her about on a regular basis, and she was getting help from every side. With a perfectly straight face, she announced to all who would listen that all her stroke damage had suddenly reappeared.

A local doctor made the statement that the only way this could happen is if she suffered another stroke. In my opinion, secondary gain is not a rational, conscious decision. More likely it is an unconscious reaction when one, who has been the pampered, babied, center of attention for a long time suddenly finds that attention waning as one recovers.

SUGGESTIONS FOR STROKE SUBJECTS

At the beginning use the "pin prick" test. If an arm or leg or both is cold and devoid of feeling (this can be tested by a gentle pin prick), proceed as follows: carefully prick shoulder or hip until you find feeling. Then take a firm, soft object (I use a tennis ball) and literally "push" feeling into arm, fingers, leg and toes. You may have to do this a couple of times. When the extremity becomes warm to touch, you have succeeded.

Using the same method, "push" strength into affected limbs.

Have subject see and feel healing light over entire body.

See and feel the light concentrating on affected parts, blood flowing freely.

Pick up ball with affected hand, eventually throw ball.

Lift ball high, slowly lower. Repeat several times.

Ask what needs to be done.

Suggest he feels nerves tingle or jump as feeling returns.

Work on cells in brain and down backbone, removing dead cells and repairing damaged cells. Healthy cells will assume duties of dead cells.

Mentally "stretch" all affected muscles.

Listen carefully to anything subject says.

Increase blood to any swollen area, elevate, suggest increased blood flow will drain any fluid collected.

Picture self as well, prior to stroke.

Warm light is "thawing out" frozen nerves and muscles.

You will sleep well tonight, and in your dreams you will see and feel light traveling over your affected parts, healing what needs to be healed. You will feel affected extremities becoming warm and realize the blood had accumulated there to nourish, relax and energize nerves and muscles.

Reinforce self-image. "You are doing this YOURSELF, no doctors, no nurses. I am merely helping you find the way. You are very proud of yourself, and of what you are doing."

Do not be afraid to improvise; use your imagination. A hypnotist is only as adept as his or her imagination.

AFTERWORD

AFTER RISKING LIFE AND LIMB searching for the entrance to the cave in the mountains above Millboro, I judiciously decided to give the Millboro story a rest. Perhaps, given time, a group of explorers more skilled in the art of spelunking will find a way into the cavern. The Millboro research has covered a span of approximately seventeen years.

As a veteran of WWII, for a while I was a member of the American Legion. One Memorial Day, I accompanied a group of veterans to a local veteran's hospital. I understand that there are many cases of phantom limb pain in V.A. hospitals. While talking to the administrator, I volunteered to spend one afternoon a week working, at no charge, with veterans in pain. Despite the fact that I should be used to it, his reaction stunned me. He was horrified that I would suggest such a thing and furthermore, the government would never stand for it for a minute. The impression I got was that he was about to bodily throw me out of the facility, so I left. A few weeks later, a friend of mine told me about her cousin, a patient at the Long Beach Veteran's Hospital who, after beseeching the doctors to perform several additional surgeries on the stump of a leg that had been amputated, finally, in desperation, shot and killed himself to escape the phantom pain that tormented him.

Many of the stories in this book were researched as much as thirty years ago. The homosexual study reinforces ideas with us today. Gay people do not want to change their orientation, do not want anyone attempting to change them. They are, however, extremely interested and curious about what it is that makes them gay. Why do they have brothers and sisters that are perfectly "normal"? The one outstanding point upon which they all agree is that the gay orientation is innate. None of them ever consciously chose to be gay.

The twin study strongly indicates to me that John Locke's theory of the "tabula rasa," that the mind is a blank slate at birth, is erroneous. In fact, throughout the thirty years I have worked with hypnosis, I am continually amazed at the interesting, sometimes colorful, weird and wonderful things that are buried deeply in all our minds—things that had to be there at birth, as none of us could have lived, in this lifetime, long enough to have amassed such a storehouse of information. Let me reiterate that this work indicates that only identical twins appear to be hiding the same past-life memories. Work with fraternal twins disclosed that they share some past lifetimes but not all.

Bringing my daughter through her birth, hearing her describe the experience step by step from the fetus' point of view was very engrossing as I was so personally involved in the entire process. I was not aware that her feet had actually started out of the birth canal and had been forced back into my body by the doctor. But I do vividly recall the reaction in the room. Suddenly all was chaos, nurses and interns rushing into the room, metal tables bearing instruments clanging into the room, frantic activity everywhere.

The "stroke" work is a concept that has been dancing about in the back of my mind for many years. When I first learned that one could direct an entranced subject to unwittingly raise a hand or arm (or foot) into the air by manipulating his autonomic nervous system, I immediately wondered if this would work with a stroke victim. Finally, I tried it and the results are as I portrayed them in the book.

Ray Conniff died very suddenly as the result of a fall. We who knew him were heartbroken to lose him so unexpectedly. He was a sweet, charming, gracious man who was, at times, humorous without even realizing it.

When he first arrived at my door, his wife, Vera, was practically carrying him. Too weak to hold a pen in order to sign the release form allowing me to use his name and photo in my book, Vera had to sign it for him.

Because of strong religious compunctions, Ray fought the hypnosis vehemently for six months. Finally, because he was making absolutely no progress, Vera insisted he let me work with him.

For the first two or three sessions, Ray fought the hypnosis. I could sense his resistance while I worked with him. During his second sessions, as I was giving him a lengthy induction, he suddenly opened his eyes and demanded, "How does God feel about this?"

Stunned, I searched for words and finally stated, "Gee, I don't know, Ray. I have not discussed it with him lately."

Another time he asked if we were offending God by doing this, and I answered that I did not think so.

Beginning the next session, I was ready for him. He obviously wanted to discuss religion so I informed him that to experience what I consider to be religion at its finest he should attend an Alcoholics Anonymous meeting.

He looked shocked for a moment, then answered, "Well, you know I am a musician and many times we played until 2:00 A.M. By the time the 'gig' was over we were all pretty well keyed up, so we would go to someone's hotel room and do a lot of drinking." He concluded his story with, "I have been a member of A.A. for forty years." The conversation continued as follows:

Me: "Do you think you were offending God by going to A.A. for help with your drinking?

Ray: "Heavens, no!"

Me: "Do you think you are offending God by coming to me for help in recovering from your stroke?"

Ray: "Heavens, no."

Me: "Fine. Let's get to work!"

There followed no more resistance, and, in my opinion, Ray was recovering very nicely when he died at the age of eighty-five.

Because the results of the work with stroke patients has been so gratifying, it is my intention to continue down this avenue. Perhaps others, paralyzed by something other than a stroke can be helped in a similar fashion. It is certainly worth looking into.

BIBLIOGRAPHY

The Powers of Hypnosis, Jean Dauven, Stein & Day, NY.

Clinical and Experimental Hypnosis, Kroger, Lippincott, Philadelphia, PA.

Hypnosis in the Relief of Pain, Hilgard & Hilgard, Kaufmann, Los Altos, CA.

New Concepts of Hypnosis, Gindes, M.D., Wilshire Book Co., N. Hollywood, CA.

Hypnotherapy, Dave Elman, Westwood Publishing Co., Los Angeles, CA.

The Autonomic Nervous System, Dr. S. Bakewell, Addenbrooke's Hospital, Cambridge, MA (from Internet).

Mesmerism in India and Its Practical Application in Surgery and Medicine, James Esdaille, 1851, Asia Educational Services, New Delhi, 1989.

ABOUT THE AUTHOR

MARGE RIEDER, PH.D., has worked in the field of experimental hypnosis for over thirty years. She has lectured throughout southern California on Past-Life Regression and conducted classes on Visual Imagery and Self-Hypnosis.

After attending Santa Ana College, she received advanced degrees from Newport University in Hypnosis and Behavior Modification. She is a graduate of the Professional Hypnosis Center in Tustin, California, is registered with the Hypnotists Examining Council, a member of the American Guild of Hypnotherapists, the American Board of Hypnotherapy, and the Association for Past Life Research and Therapies. She has published a number of articles in magazines and professional journals as well as two previous books: *Mission to Millboro* and *Return to Millboro.*

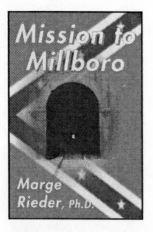

Mission to Millboro

A Study in Group Reincarnation

Marge Rieder, Ph.D.

ISBN: 0-931892-59-7, 208 pages, 43 photos,
5.5 x 8.5, paper, $13.00

Not one, but more than thirty-five people have been identified, most of them from around Lake Elsinore, California, who, under hypnosis, can recall in graphic detail, life in the same little town in Virginia during the American Civil War! Using the information gained during the hypnotherapy sessions, Dr. Rieder enthralls us by showing the secret tunnels and hideaways she uncovered while on her expeditions to Millboro. She skillfully reconstructs the suspenseful stories of love, tragedy and espionage that echo through the past and impact the present.

"A must-read for the curious and skeptical alike."
—**Pyramid Books**

*"Dr. Marge Rieder skillfully combines an intriguing spy story worthy of John Le Carré with well-developed psychological research into how the past, even though consciously forgotten, continues to influence our lives today. **Mission to Millboro** is a thoroughly enjoyable book. I couldn't put it down."*
—**Chet B. Snow, Ph.D.**, *Mass Dreams of the Future*

"The Millboro case is one of the most fascinating examples of group reincarnation I have ever read. After personally meeting three of the subjects, I am even more impressed with their story."
—**Bruce Goldberg, D.D.S., M.S.**, *The Search for Grace*

Blue Dolphin Publishing
Orders: 1-800-643-0765 • Web: www.bluedolphinpublishing.com

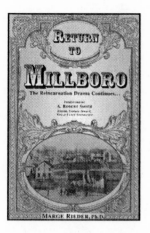

Return to Millboro

The Reincarnation Drama Continues

Marge Rieder, Ph.D.

ISBN: 0-931892-28-7, 256 pages, 40 photos, 5.5 x 8.5, paper, $14.95

The dramatic story that unfolded in Dr. Rieder's first book, *Mission to Millboro,* is revisited in this intriguing story, as more people are discovered, under hypnosis, to have memories from Millboro. After several trips to the present-day Millboro, Dr. Rieder shares her impressions and the detective work involved in finding evidence to prove the uncanny accuracy of these centuries-old memories.

"Marge Rieder has done it again! **Return to Millboro** *is even more compelling than its predecessor, as her cast of Civil War characters expands to include prehistoric Indians, runaway slaves, and the underground railroad."*
— **Chet B. Snow. Ph.D.**, *Mass Dreams of the Future*

"The entranced Edgar Cayce spoke of group reincarnation; Marge Rieder has demonstrated it! In this sequel to **Mission to Millboro***, she presents the conclusion of an air-tight case for group rebirth, proving it beyond a reasonable doubt. The evidence, both internal and external, is overwhelming. ... An extraordinary piece of past-life research, the best of its kind to date."*
— **George Schwimmer, Ph.D.**, *The Search for David*

Blue Dolphin Publishing
Orders: 1-800-643-0765 • Web: www.bluedolphinpublishing.com

Printed in the United States
1396300001B/385-426